McGRAW-HILL'S

Pocket Guide
to Chest X-rays

M000280526

This book is dedicated to
Joshua Tamone (1987–2003)
... who will be remembered for his smile ...

McGRAW-HILL'S

Pocket Guide to Chest X-rays

Greg Briggs MBBS, FRCR
Senior Staff Radiologist
Royal North Shore Hospital, Sydney
Senior Clinical Lecturer
The University of Sydney

*The **McGraw·Hill** Companies*

Sydney New York San Francisco Auckland
Bangkok Bogotá Caracas Hong Kong
Kuala Lumpur Lisbon London Madrid
Mexico City Milan New Delhi San Juan
Seoul Singapore Taipei Toronto

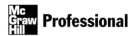

National Library of Australia Cataloguing-in-Publication data:

Briggs, Greg.
McGraw-Hill's pocket guide to chest X-Rays.

Bibliography.
Includes index.
ISBN 0 074 71336 1.

1.Thoracic radiography. 2. Diagnosis, Radioscopic. 3. Chest—Diseases—Diagnosis. I. Title.
617.540747

Published in Australia by
McGraw-Hill Australia Pty Ltd
Level 2, 82 Waterloo Road, North Ryde NSW 2113
Acquisitions Editor: Meiling Voon
Production Editor: Sybil Kesteven
Editor: Carolyn Pike
Editorial Assistant: Thu Nguyen
Proofreader: Joy Window
Indexer: Glenda Browne
Cover design: Lara Scott
Illustrator: Alan Laver, Shelly Communications
Image preparation: Peter Freeman, Freedom Graphics
Typeset in 8.5/11 pt Sabon by Jan Schmoeger/Designpoint
Printed on 80 gsm matt art by Pantech Limited, Hong Kong.

The *McGraw·Hill* Companies

Contents

Notice

Medicine is an ever-changing science. As new research and clinical experience broaden our knowledge, changes in treatment and drug therapy are required. The editors and the publisher of this work have checked with sources believed to be reliable in their efforts to provide information that is complete and generally in accord with the standards accepted at the time of publication. However, in view of the possibility of human error or changes in medical sciences, neither the editors, nor the publisher, nor any other party who has been involved in the preparation or publication of this work warrants that the information contained herein is in every respect accurate or complete. Readers are encouraged to confirm the information contained herein with other sources. For example, and in particular, readers are advised to check the product information sheet included in the package of each drug they plan to administer to be certain that the information contained in this book is accurate and that changes have not been made in the recommended dose or in the contraindications for administration. This recommendation is of particular importance in connection with new or infrequently used drugs.

Preface

In spite of ever-improving sophisticated and advanced medical imaging technology, the chest radiograph remains the most common medical imaging procedure performed. It provides an easily obtained source of information on the heart and lungs—the 'engine room' of the body.

The interpretation of the chest radiograph requires a basic understanding of radiography, a knowledge of chest anatomy and pathology, and a search for radiological clues. This has formed the basis for the chapter layout.

Radiological signs that are seen in computed tomography are included in Appendix 1 because of the overlap with plain film findings and to provide a comprehensive list.

I hope that this pocket guide will provide a good introduction to chest radiology to novice radiologists, chest physicians and cardiothoracic surgeons.

Acknowledgments

Firstly, I am grateful to Anne Streeter for her dedication and helpfulness in typing the complete manuscript from my notes and many changes.

I am thankful to Dr Anne Miller for her contribution of Figures 3.3, 4.2 and 4.6.

I appreciate Professor WSC Hare's permission to reproduce Figure 3.7 which is from his book *Clinical Radiology for Medical Students and Health Practitioners*.

The publishing team at McGraw-Hill deserve praise for their professionalism and initiation of this project.

Finally, I wish to acknowledge my radiological and clinical colleagues, radiographers, junior medical staff, medical students, nurses and paramedical staff who have stimulated my interest in chest radiology.

Glossary

The glossary is a list of definitions of terms used in chest radiology. Those terms defined in Appendix 1, Signs in Thoracic Radiology, have not been repeated here. The following references give a comprehensive list of recommendations:

- Tuddenham WJ. Glossary of terms for thoracic radiology: recommendations of the Nomenclature Committee of the Fleischner Society. *AJR* 1984;143:509–17.
- Austin JHM, Muller NL, Friedman PJ et al. Glossary of terms for CT of the lungs: recommendations of the Nomenclature Committee of the Fleischner Society. *Radiology* 1996;200:327–31.
- Webb RW, Muller NL, Naidich DP. Illustrated glossary in high-resolution computed tomography terms. In: High resolution CT of the lung. 3rd edn. Baltimore: Lippincott, Williams & Wilkins, 2001: 599–618.

air bronchogram The bronchus is visible as an air-filled structure surrounded by consolidated or collapsed lung.

airspace The gas-containing part of the lung, including the respiratory bronchioles, but excluding the purely conducting airways.

air-trapping Abnormal retention of air within part of a lung on expiration as a result of airway obstruction.

airway Collective term for air-conducting passages from the larynx to the terminal bronchiole.

architectural distortion Abnormal displacement of lung structures due to lung disease.

atelectasis Collapse and volume loss are synonymous terms.

attenuation (*verb*: attenuate) The process by which the energy of an X-ray beam is reduced as it passes through matter. This reduction is by either absorption or scattering.

bleb A small gas space inside the visceral pleura usually occurring after surgery. Blebs are smaller than bullae and can cause pneumothoraces.

bronchial wall thickening Oedema, inflammatory or neoplastic cells infiltrate the peribronchial interstitial space.

bronchiectasis Bronchial dilatation which often has associated bronchial wall thickening.

bulla (*plural*: bullae; *adjective*: bullous) An emphysematous space which normally has a very thin wall and communicates with the bronchial tree. The bulla is more than 1 cm in size and, if ruptured, can cause a pneumothorax.

calcification (*adjective*: calcified) Deposition of calcium salts within a structure rendering it visible on X-ray examination.

cavity Thick-walled space containing air, or air and fluid, with an air–fluid level.

consolidation Filling of the airspaces with abnormal material, such as transudate, exudate, cells or protein. Consolidated lung characteristically appears dense and shows the bronchi as air-filled tubular structures (see Air bronchogram sign, Appendix 1) but obscures the underlying vessels.

cor pulmonale In the presence of severe lung disease the right heart becomes dilated. The central pulmonary arteries become dilated because of the pulmonary hypertension.

cyst Thin-walled space containing either air or fluid.

density General non-specific term for any area of whiteness on the chest radiograph.

end-stage lung This is the final common appearance of a number of chronic infiltrative lung diseases and is characterised by the presence of fibrosis, alveolar loss, bronchiolectasis and disruption of normal lung architecture.

flail chest A chest wall injury that disturbs the mechanics of ventilation because of the abnormal mobility. It occurs when there are more than five contiguous single fractures or when there are three or more double rib fractures. Typically associated with lung injury and possibly extrathoracic injury.

ground-glass opacity Hazy increase in lung density.

hilum (*plural*: hila; *adjective*: hilar) The hilum is an imprecisely defined anatomical region which is the junction area between the mediastinum and lung.

interstitium (*adjective*: interstitial) The loose connective tissue that forms the structure for the lungs. It includes the connective tissues around the bronchi and vessels and the interlobular septae. It is not normally visible radiographically but thickens with disease processes.

kVp The peak kilovoltage across an X-ray tube. A higher kVp produces higher energy X-rays.

lucency (*adjective*: lucent) An area of blackness on the radiograph due to the transmission of X-rays through matter. (*synonyms*: translucency, transradiancy)

mA (milliampere/second) The amount of current through an X-ray tube. It determines the quantity of the X-rays generated to produce an image.

mass A discrete opacity > 3 cm in size.

mycetoma Fungus ball.

nodule A discrete opacity < 3 cm in size.

nosocomial pneumonia A general term for hospital-acquired pneumonia.

opacity Synonym for density.

pneumatocoele Thin-walled, transient, gas-filled space in the lungs; seen with staphylococcal and *Pneumocystis carinii* pneumonia; also seen after trauma and hydrocarbon pneumonia. It is presumed that it is a tension cyst due to obstruction of a bronchiole.

pneumomediastinum Air present in the mediastinum outside the oesophagus and tracheobronchial tree.

pneumopericardium Air present in the pericardial space.

pneumothorax Free gas in the pleural space (i.e. between the parietal and visceral pleura). It may be modified by the prefixes hydro-, pyo-, haemo- and chylo-.

reticular shadowing Fine, medium or coarse irregular linear opacities due to interstitial thickening.

tomogram A special radiograph in which one plane is in focus with the planes above and below blurred out. It is achieved by moving the X-ray tube and cassette in different directions during exposure.

Valsalva manoeuvre Forced expiration against a closed glottis. This produces an increase in thoracic pressure.

Common abbreviations and acronyms

ABMA	antibasement membrane antibody
ABPA	allergic bronchopulmonary aspergillosis
AIDS	acquired immunodeficiency syndrome
AILD	angioimmunoblastic lymphadenopathy
AIP	acute interstitial pneumonia
AMBER	advanced multiple beam equalisation radiography
ANCA	antineutrophil cytoplasmic antibodies
AP	anteroposterior
ARDS	adult respiratory distress syndrome
ASD	atrial septal defect
AVF	arteriovenous fistula
BAC	bronchioalveolar carcinoma
BAL	bronchoalveolar lavage
BALT	bronchus-associated lymphoma tumour (see MALT)
BCG	bacille Calmette-Guérin
BHL	bilateral hilar lymphadenopathy
BIP	bronchiolitis obliterans and diffuse interstitial pneumonia
BOOP	bronchiolitis obliterans with organising pneumonia
CAL	chronic airways limitation
CAT	computerised axial tomography
CCF	congestive cardiac failure
CD4	this is a type of T lymphocyte using the cluster of differentiation (CD) classification

CDS	ciliary dyskinesia syndrome
CECT	contrast-enhanced computed tomography
CF	cystic fibrosis
CFA	crytogenic fibrosing alveolitis
CID	cytomegalic inclusion disease
CIP	chronic interstitial pneumonitis
CLL	chronic lymphocytic leukemia
CMV	cytomegalovirus
COAD	chronic obstructive airways disease
COP	cryptogenic organising pneumonia
COPD	chronic obstructive pulmonary disease
CREST	calcinosis, Raynaud's syndrome, oesophageal dysmotility, sclerodactyly and telangiectasis
CT	computed tomography
CTPA	computed tomographic pulmonary angiography
CTR	cardiothoracic ratio
CWP	coal workers' pneumoconiosis
CXR	chest X-ray (chest radiograph)
DAD	diffuse alveolar damage
DCS	dyskinetic cilia syndrome
DD	differential diagnosis
DIC	disseminated intravascular coagulation
DIP	desquamative interstitial pneumonia
DPH	diffuse pulmonary haemorrhage
DVT	deep venous/vein thrombosis
EAA	extrinsic allergic alveolitis
ECG	electrocardiogram
EG	eosinophilic granuloma
ESL	end-stage lung
ETT	endotracheal tube
GBM	glomerular basement membrane
GGO	ground-glass opacity
GIP	giant cell interstitial pneumonia
HIV	human immunodeficiency virus
HP	hypersensitivity pneumonia
HRCT	high-resolution computed tomography
HU	Hounsfield units
ICC	intercostal catheter
II	image intensifier

ILD	interstitial lung disease
INH	isonicotinic acid hydrazide (isoniazid)
IPF	idiopathic pulmonary fibrosis
IPH	idiopathic pulmonary haemosiderosis
IVC	inferior vena cava
LAM	lymphangioleiomyomatosis
LDH	lactate dehydrogenase
LIP	lymphocytic interstitial pneumonia
LVRS	lung volume reduction surgery
MAC	same as MAI
MAI	*Mycobacterium avium-intracellulare*
MALT	mucosa-associated lymphoid tissue
MOT	*Mycobacterium* other than tuberculosis
MRI	magnetic resonance imaging
NF	neurofibromatosis
NSIP	non-specific interstitial pneumonia
NTM	non-tuberculous *Mycobacterium*
PA	posteroanterior
PACS	picture archiving and communication system
PAH	pulmonary arterial hypertension
PAP	pulmonary alveolar proteinosis
PAWP	pulmonary artery wedge pressures
PCP	*Pneumocystis carinii* pneumonia
PDA	patent ductus arteriosus
PE	pulmonary embolism
PEEP	positive end-expiratory pressure
PET	positron emission tomography
PIE (adult)	pulmonary infiltrate with eosinophilia
PIE (neonate)	pulmonary interstitial emphysema
PLCH	pulmonary Langerhans cell histiocytosis
PMF	progressive massive fibrosis
PNET	primitive neuroectodermal tumour
PPD	purified protein derivative of tuberculin
PTLD	post-transplant lymphoproliferative disorder
RB	respiratory bronchiolitis, as in RB-ILD
RML	right middle lobe
RMLS	right middle lobe syndrome
RSV	respiratory syncytial virus
SARS	severe acute respiratory syndrome

SCUBA	self-contained underwater breathing apparatus
SIADH	syndrome of inappropriate secretion of antidiuretic hormone
SLE	systemic lupus erythematosus
SPN	solitary pulmonary nodule
SVC	superior vena cava
TAPVR	total anomalous pulmonary venous return
TB	tuberculosis
TIPS	transjugular intrahepatic portosystemic shunt
TNM	tumour–node–metastasis staging system
TOE	transoesophageal echocardiography
TOF	tracheo-oesophageal fistula
TS	tuberous sclerosis
UIP	usual interstitial pneumonia
US	ultrasound
VATER	vertebral/vascular, anal, cardiac, tracheo-oesophageal, renal/radial anomalies
VATS	video-assisted thorascopic surgery
V/Q	ventilation/perfusion isotope scan
VSD	ventricular septal defect

Chapter 1

Introduction to techniques

Chest radiograph

X-rays were discovered in 1895 by Conrad Roentgen, a German physicist. They are a form of energy and are part of the electromagnetic spectrum, lying between gamma rays and ultraviolet light. They are produced when a stream of electrons in a vacuum tube passes from the cathode and strikes the anode. Because of their short wavelength, X-rays can penetrate materials that do not transmit visible light. However, different degrees of absorption and penetration of the X-rays occur as they pass in a straight line through the body because of the varying tissue densities. The X-rays exiting from the body can expose photosensitive film to allow us to record these different densities within the body. For example, very little absorption occurs in the lungs and the X-rays pass through to expose the film black, whereas the bones absorb the X-rays and, with reduced exposure, the film is white. If the lung airspaces become filled in disease processes, the denser or consolidated lungs appear whiter on the radiograph.

The plain chest radiograph, colloquially called the chest X-ray (CXR), is the most commonly performed imaging procedure in most radiology practices. The standard frontal chest radiograph is with the beam of X-rays in a posteroanterior (PA) direction relative to the patient. The front of the patient is against the film cassette with the X-ray tube about 2–4 m behind. The radiographer centres the beam on the T4 vertebra and instructs patients to put their wrists on their hips to displace the scapulae laterally so as not to obscure the lung fields.

Conventional chest radiography (60–80 kVp) has been improved using higher energy X-rays produced with a higher kilovoltage. With a high kilovoltage technique (120–140 kVp), the bony structures appear less dense and permit better visualisation of the mediastinum and more of the lung parenchyma. The only disadvantage is the reduced visualisation of calcific densities in the lungs. A grid or air gap is used to reduce scatter radiation exposing the film.

The ideal studies are the PA erect and left lateral view radiographs obtained on full inspiration, so that maximal lung volume is visualised.

Many ill patients need to be radiographed in bed with anteroposterior (AP) projections. These views produce reduced diagnostic information but fortunately are only needed to exclude or confirm major disease processes or are only performed to evaluate line or tube placement (see Fig. 1.1).

Fig. 1.1 (a) Posteroanterior (PA) versus (b) anteroposterior (AP) views of the chest

Wherever possible the frontal film should ideally be a PA study. Even in the X-ray department, the patient may be unable to stand for a PA view and an AP view is performed. Not all AP views are the same technique and therefore are of varying quality. They could be departmental or 'mobile', erect or supine.

The AP mobile film should be used for ill patients who have difficulty moving and where space is limited at the bedside. Because of the longer exposure times on the AP film and the expected poorer centring, the film quality is not as good. Fortunately, the AP film is good for showing lines and catheters and gross pleural and pulmonary disease but magnification spoils assessment of cardiac size. The supine AP film is restricted to very ill patients or those patients who cannot sit up. The AP supine film will be less helpful than the AP erect film in showing pleural effusions.

It is mandatory for the radiograph to be labelled as 'AP' by the radiographer. If such labelling is missing, clues include the position of the scapulae, shape of the ribs and the smaller visible lung volumes.

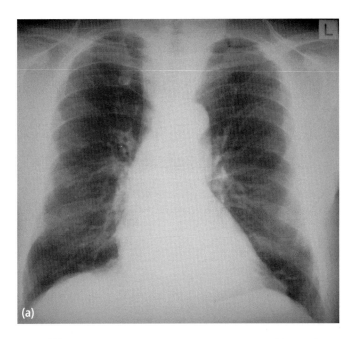

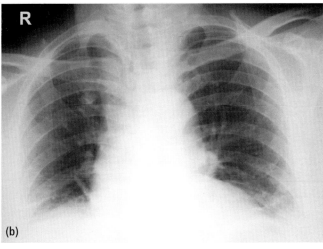

Other projections include supine expiratory, oblique, lordotic, penetrated or lateral decubitus views (see Table 1.1 and Fig. 1.2).

The X-ray film is protected within a cassette, which also contains intensification screens. The intensification screens produce light to augment the X-ray exposure of the photosensitive film and allow a reduction in the amount of irradiation required for the patient. Recent improvements are faster film emulsions, faster intensification screens, wide-latitude film and asymmetric film–screen combinations.

The technical challenge in chest radiography is the big contrast difference between the lungs (air density) and the mediastinum. The mediastinum attenuates (absorbs) the X-rays about ten times more than the lungs. The *advanced multiple beam equalisation radiography* system (AMBER) uses an electronic feedback system to enable a slit beam of X-rays to produce a more uniformly exposed chest radiograph. This AMBER technique evens out the wide contrast differences between the lungs and mediastinum to provide a better image.

Further technical improvements are digital systems that use selenium-based, flat-panel detectors or storage phosphor systems with either hard-copy viewing or soft-copy viewing on a *cathode ray tube* (CRT) monitor. The monitors with a 2000×2000 matrix (pixel size, 0.2 mm) are better.

The digital image is simply a representation of a picture as a two-dimensional array of numbers. Each number represents a single picture element (pixel) in the image. The value of each pixel defines the brightness, or greyscale value, of that point in the image.

Table 1.1 Radiographic views	
Projections/techniques	**Indication**
PA	Varied
AP (department or mobile) (erect or supine)	Ill patient
Expiration	Pneumothorax, air-trapping
Oblique	Rib fracture, pleural plaques
Lordotic	Apical and middle lobe disease
Lateral decubitus	Pleural effusion, pneumothorax
Lateral shoot-through	Pneumothorax

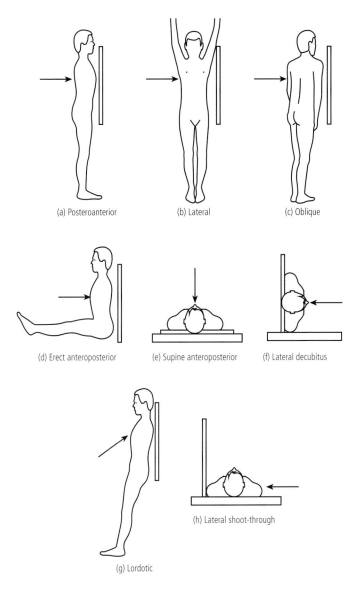

(a) Posteroanterior

(b) Lateral

(c) Oblique

(d) Erect anteroposterior

(e) Supine anteroposterior

(f) Lateral decubitus

(g) Lordotic

(h) Lateral shoot-through

Fig. 1.2 Chest radiographic projections

The digital systems have advantages in image acquisition, transmission, display and storage. The digital data can be used in *picture archiving and communication systems* (PACS), that is, the retrieval and transmission of the image over telephone lines.

Radiation dose

In modern chest radiography during a routine PA exposure, the lungs receive about 150 μGy (15 millirad) of radiation, the gonads about 10 μGy (1 millirad) and the skin entry dose is 500 μGy (50 millirad). The probability of a fatal cancer being induced in an individual patient from a single frontal radiograph is estimated at one per million.

In computed tomography (CT) the dose is higher by a factor of 100 and is equivalent to the background radiation that people are exposed to each year.

Fluoroscopy

Fluoroscopy is the process of viewing on a monitor a real-time image produced by a continuous, low power X-ray beam. The X-ray beam passes through the body and stimulates an image intensifier (II), which converts the signal into a television image. This method is used to screen the diaphragmatic movements and to aid arteriography and interventional procedures, such as lung tumour biopsy.

Computed tomography

CT is a non-invasive diagnostic technique that provides more information than the standard radiograph but uses more radiation. The images are more sensitive in detecting abnormalities and provide better anatomic detail.

A narrow, collimated beam of revolving X-rays is transmitted through the body to a ring of detectors to give a cross-sectional image. The density of small volumes (voxels) in the body can be calculated with computers from the multiple projections. The CT image itself is composed of a matrix of picture elements (pixels).

The density of each voxel is measured in Hounsfield units (HU). The reference value for water is 0 HU and for air is −1000 HU.

In spiral/helical scanning, the patient is moved through the CT gantry on the sliding table top at a constant rate while being scanned. The variable factors are the speed of travel, slice thickness and scan length. The ratio of the table movement occurring during a complete tube rotation to the slice thickness is referred to as the 'pitch'. The data can be rapidly acquired on a single breath hold. Multidetector scanners allow even faster data acquisition, greater anatomic coverage, optimal contrast enhancement and improved spatial resolution.

High-resolution CT scanning (HRCT) shows fine detail of the lung by using thin sections (1 mm) and a high-frequency spatial reconstruction algorithm.

Magnetic resonance imaging (MRI)

MRI is a non-invasive diagnostic technique that uses external magnetic fields and radiofrequency waves to produce an image. When the patient lies in an MRI scanner, the hydrogen nuclei in water and fat molecules within the body become aligned with the magnetic field. When a special pulse of radiofrequency energy is applied, the nuclei are initially flipped but then return to their original state. The change in energy level and spin, which are different for various tissues, are measured and converted by computers into a greyscale image.

In the thorax, the main uses are for assessment of apical lung tumours, aortic dissection and cardiac motion.

Isotope scanning

Isotope scanning uses various radioactive labelled agents to detect abnormalities. The main nuclear medicine studies in the thorax are:
- ventilation and perfusion scanning (*V/Q* scan), using radioactive gas and technetium-99 albumin microspheres to detect pulmonary emboli
- myocardial infarct imaging with thallium-201
- technetium-labelled phosphonates for bony secondary deposits
- positron emission tomography (PET)—the uptake of the radiopharmaceutical fluoro-2-deoxy-D-glucose (FDG) is used to help stage lung carcinoma.

Ultrasound

Ultrasound is sound waves with a frequency above the human hearing range. Ultrasound waves are produced by a piezoelectric crystal in the transducer probe, which also detects their returning signal. The echo signal is converted into an electrical signal and this is subsequently processed into a greyscale picture.

Ultrasound is helpful in localising pleural effusions to facilitate drainage. Doppler ultrasound can be used to assess blood flow velocities and is a non-invasive technique of diagnosing deep vein thrombosis.

Pulmonary angiography

In pulmonary angiography, a catheter is passed via a peripheral vein, usually the right common femoral vein, through the right side of the heart to selectively catheterise the pulmonary artery. The injected contrast shows the pulmonary arterial and venous circulations. Pulmonary angiography is the 'gold standard' for detection of pulmonary emboli.

Bronchial angiography

Selective catheterisation of the bronchial arteries may be required to demonstrate the site and cause of haemoptysis. This study is needed before bronchial artery embolisation.

Interventional procedures

- Lung biopsy. Under fluoroscopic or CT guidance, a needle can be inserted into a pulmonary, pleural or mediastinal mass. The aspirated material is used for cytological and microbiological analysis.
- Abscess and emphysema drainage. A catheter can be introduced percutaneously under imaging guidance to drain pus collections.
- Pleural fluid aspiration. A needle can be inserted into small effusions under ultrasound guidance and a specimen aspirated for analysis.
- Bronchial artery embolisation. Embolic material, such as coils (cotton-coated metallic threads), can be used to occlude bleeding bronchial arteries caused by bronchiectasis.

Chapter 2
Basic radiologic anatomy

A basic knowledge of chest anatomy is needed to understand the appearances on the chest X-ray (CXR). In CXR interpretation, the first decision is whether the appearances are normal or not. Only with a sound knowledge of the radiologic anatomy can the interpretation proceed. With experience, the radiologist becomes aware of differences in anatomy due to body habitus, degree of inspiration and position of the patient.

Chest anatomy

Airways

The normal adult trachea is 1.5–1.8 cm wide, mid-line in the lower neck and deviates slightly to the right as it lies on the right side of the aortic arch. In cadaveric anatomy and on expiration the carina lies at the T4 level. On inspiration the carina will move inferiorly to the T6 level. In adults, the right main bronchus has a steeper angle than does the left but the angles are symmetrical in children.

The adult right main bronchus is 2.5 cm long and is 25° from the vertical, whereas the left main bronchus is 4.5 cm long and 45° from the vertical. The difference is due to the early origin of the right upper lobe bronchus (see Fig. 2.1). The intermediate bronchus continues for 3 cm before dividing into the middle and right lower lobe bronchi.

The more vertical orientation of the right main bronchus explains why an over-advanced endotracheal tube enters it and can obstruct the right upper lobe bronchus or left lung (see Figs 2.2 and 4.5b).

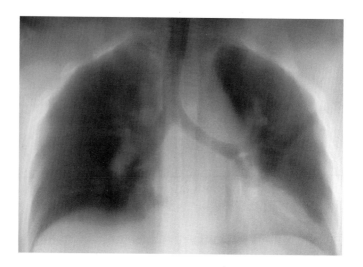

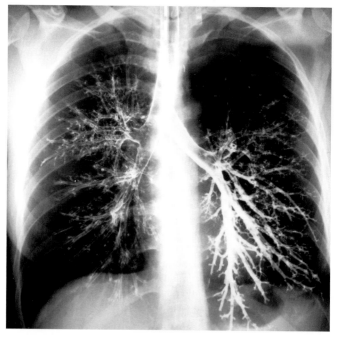

Fig. 2.1 Tracheal tomogram

The conventional tomogram has been produced by movement of the X-ray tube and film so that only the plane 'in focus' is not blurred. In this case, the anatomy of the trachea and main bronchi is well seen. Please note the azygos vein, prominent with the patient supine, at the right tracheobronchial angle coming forward to drain into the superior vena cava (SVC).

Fig. 2.2 Bronchial anatomy

Bronchograms are an outmoded imaging technique where special iodine-based contrast media were instilled into the bronchial tree. With tipping and gravity, all the segmental bronchi were able to be outlined. These studies were useful to demonstrate bronchiectasis.

Please note the asymmetry in the main right and left bronchi with the right upper lobe bronchus arising early.

The lobar bronchi divide into segmental bronchi to supply the corresponding lung segments.

Lungs

Each lung is divided into lobes by fissures, which are reflections of the visceral pleura: the right lung has three lobes—upper, middle and lower; the left lung has two lobes—upper and lower. The lungs are further subdivided into ten segments on the right and eight segments on the left. On the left side, the equivalent of the middle lobe is the lingular segments of the upper lobe (see Fig. 2.3).

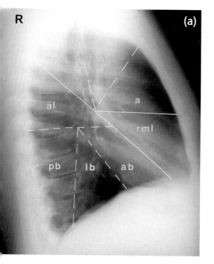

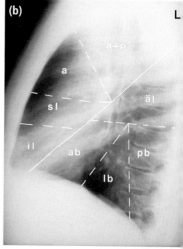

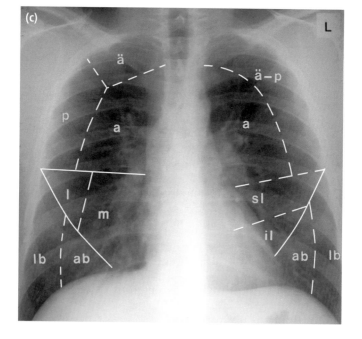

Fig. 2.3 Lung segments: (a) right lateral view; (b) left lateral view; (c) PA view

The lung segments fit together in the lung like a three-dimensional jigsaw. They correspond to the bronchial divisions. There are ten segments in the right lung and eight segments in the left lung. The numbering system is seen in the key. For example, the bronchus in the apical segment of the lower lobe is called B6. The lingular segments of the left upper lobe correspond to the middle lobe; there is no left medial basal segment as this space is occupied by the heart; the apical and posterior segments of the left upper lobe are fused.

Please note that the oblique fissures pass from about 4 cm behind the cardiophrenic angle through the hilum to T4.

Key:

Right upper lobe			Left upper lobe		
B1	ä	apical	B1, B3	ä-p	apicoposterior
B2	a	anterior	B2	a	anterior
B3	p	posterior			
Right middle lobe					
B4	l	lateral	B4	sl	superior lingula
B5	m	medial	B5	il	inferior lingula
Right lower lobe			**Left lower lobe**		
B6	äl	apical lower	B6	äl	apical lower
B7	mb	medial basal			
B8	ab	anterior basal	B7, B8	ab	anteromedial basal
B9	lb	lateral basal	B9	lb	lateral basal
B10	pb	posterior basal	B10	pb	posterior basal

The fissures are incomplete in the majority of patients but are important landmarks in lobar anatomy. However, the fissures are an inconstant finding, with the horizontal fissure only seen in 50% of chest radiographs.

The major interlobular fissure on each side passes obliquely as a plane from '4 to 4', that is, from 4 cm behind the anterior costophrenic angle through the hilum to the T4 level (as seen on the lateral view). In the right lung, the major fissure separates the lower lobe from the upper and middle lobes; in the left lung, it separates the upper and lower lobes. The horizontal fissure (or minor fissure) separates the middle lobe from the upper lobe. It lies at the level of the fourth costal cartilage and contacts the lateral chest wall near the axillary portion of the right sixth rib.

For convenience, the lung fields can be divided into upper, mid and lower zones. The upper zones lie above the level of the second costal cartilage; the mid-zones between the levels of the second and fourth costal cartilages; and the lower zones below the level of the fourth costal cartilage. The apices lie above the clavicles.

Lung parenchyma

The bronchial tree continues dividing into smaller and smaller bronchi until they lose their cartilage and become bronchioles. The terminal bronchiole is the last conducting structure. Beyond the terminal bronchioles lie the respiratory bronchioles, the alveolar ducts, alveolar sacs and alveoli—the gas-exchanging units of the lung.

The *acinus* is that portion of the lung distal to the terminale broncole, comprising the respiratory bronchioles, alveolar ducts, alveolar sacs and alveoli; it is about 5 mm in diameter.

Several acini are grouped together into a *secondary pulmonary lobule*, which is about 2 cm in diameter and polyhedral in shape. The secondary pulmonary lobules are separated from each other by connective tissue (interlobular septa). The secondary pulmonary lobule is, therefore, the smallest discrete portion of lung surrounded by connective tissue septa. The interlobular septa contain the lymphatics and venules. Thickening of the septa is seen as Kerley B lines.

In the centre of each secondary pulmonary lobule are the bronchovascular bundles, which are made up of the preterminal bronchiole and its accompanying artery.

The primary pulmonary lobule of Miller consists of all the alveolar ducts, alveolar sacs and alveoli distal to the last respiratory bronchiole. This unit is of no practical radiographic significance.

Pulmonary vessels

The pulmonary arteries extend in a tree-like manner from the hilum to the lungs (see Fig. 2.4). These branching, blood-filled band opacities (lung markings) are well seen against the air-filled lung. The veins drain back to the left atrium. In the upper lobes the vessels have a vertical orientation with the veins lateral to the arteries. In the lower lobe, the veins have a horizontal course as they drain into the left atrium, whereas arteries in the lower lobe lie more vertically. The vertical descending veins in the upper lobe add to the density of the upper portions of the hila, whereas the veins in the lower lobe contribute to the density of the lower portions of the hila. On computed tomography (CT), the anatomy of the ostia of the four pulmonary veins draining into the left atrium is of increasing interest to facilitate the radiofrequency ablation of ectopic foci.

On the erect radiograph film, the diameters of the vessels increase from the apices to the bases. The vessels in the first anterior intercostal space should not exceed 3 mm. As seen on the erect CXR, the vessels to the lower zones appear larger. Most of the ventilation and perfusion occurs in the lower zones. When the person is horizontal, equalisation of the flow occurs, with enlargement of the vessels to the upper zones. Pulmonary circulation values are shown in Table 2.1.

Hila

The hila are the imprecisely defined junctions between the mediastinal structures and the lungs. Their densities are mainly due to the pulmonary arteries but the pulmonary veins, lymph nodes and bronchi also contribute.

Table 2.1 Pulmonary circulation values	
	Value
Volume	450–600 mL (about 10% of total blood volume)
Mean arterial pressure	15 mmHg
Mean venous pressure	5 mmHg
Flow at rest	5 L/min
Flow at maximal exercise	20 L/min
Lung height	30 cm

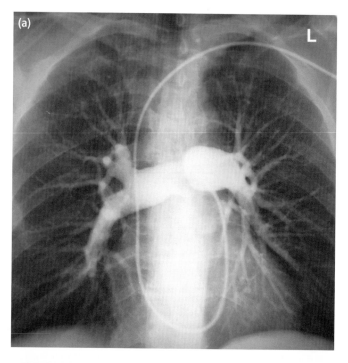

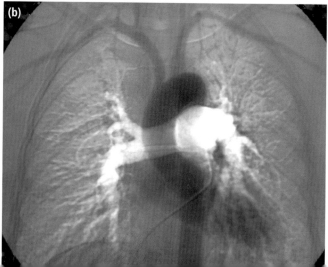

The right hilum is in the shape of a V turned on its side and lies 1–2 cm below the height of the left hilum. The left hilum is higher and has a squarer shape.

The critical fact in understanding hilar anatomy is that the left pulmonary artery arches over the left main bronchus to descend posterolateral to the left lower lobe bronchus, whereas the right pulmonary artery passes anterior to the main bronchus and intermediate bronchus, with early origin of the right upper lobe artery at the hilum.

Diaphragm

The diaphragm separates the thoracic and abdominal cavities. The anterior portion of the left hemidiaphragm is obscured by the heart but the other portions are outlined by the adjacent aerated lung. The hemidiaphragm on each side is a domed structure. The height of the curve is about 2.5 cm.

On the inspiratory frontal film, the apex of the hemidiaphragm should pass as low as the sixth costal cartilage level or the tenth to eleventh rib posteriorly. In thin young athletic patients, the level of the diaphragm will pass more inferiorly and should not be interpreted as 'over-inflation'.

The right hemidiaphragm is 2 cm higher than the left in most patients. In 10% of patients the two domes lie at the same level.

In the posteroanterior (PA) projection, the posterior lung base is hidden below the dome of the diaphragm. The lateral film shows the hemidiaphragms as well as the whole of the lung bases, including the posterior costophrenic angles.

◄ —————————————————————————————————————

Fig. 2.4 Pulmonary artery anatomy: (a) pulmonary angiogram; (b) digital subtraction angiogram

(a) A catheter has been introduced into the main pulmonary artery via a left arm catheter. The pulmonary arteries have been demonstrated with a contrast injection.

   At the right hilum, the right main pulmonary artery is dividing and lying anterior to the right main bronchus. The left pulmonary artery passes up and over the left main bronchus. The branches then radiate out into the lung fields.

(b) A catheter has been introduced from the femoral vein. It passes up the inferior vena cava (IVC), across the right atrium, tricuspid valve and right ventricle to the main pulmonary artery.

   The digital subtraction technology has helped in showing the anatomical relationship between the aorta and pulmonary arteries.

Partial eventration is when a membrane replaces part of the muscle layer and is seen as a smooth hump.

Mediastinum

The mediastinum separates the two pleural cavities and lungs, extending from the cervicothoracic junction above to the diaphragm below and from the sternum in front to the vertebral column behind. It contains a number of structures, including the heart, great vessels, trachea, oesophagus, lymph nodes, thoracic duct and mediastinal fat. Figure 2.5 shows the margins of the mediastinum.

The aortic knuckle is the junction of the aortic arch and descending aorta. It produces a characteristic configuration above the hilum on the left margin of the superior mediastinum where it is outlined by the apicoposterior segment of the left upper lobe.

The thymus is relatively large in the first three years, filling much of the anterior mediastinal space. Only during this time is it visible as a mediastinal structure on the frontal CXR (see Sail sign, Appendix 1). It grows slightly until puberty (see Fig. 2.6) and, after the teenage years, atrophies and undergoes fatty replacement. The thymus maintains cell-mediated immune responses by producing T lymphocytes.

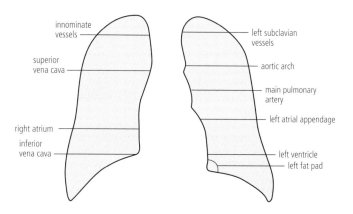

Fig. 2.5 Lateral margins of the mediastinum

Mediastinal spaces

The *pretracheal space* is explored by surgeons in transcervical mediastinoscopy in the diagnostic work-up of bronchogenic carcinoma. Lymph nodes here are amenable to biopsy. Remember that 17% of normal-appearing lymph nodes in this space may have microscopic metastases.

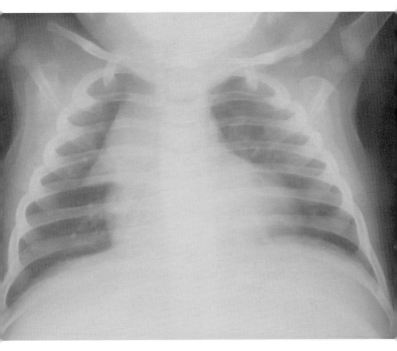

Fig. 2.6 Thymus in a neonate: AP view

In the normal neonate, the thymus often causes a triangular sail shadow, usually on the right upper mediastinum. It needs to be recognised as different from right upper lobe consolidation by its well-defined vertical lateral border; its sharp inferior angle is not seen in encapsulated pleural effusion.

Besides this sail sign, other signs to distinguish the thymus are the spinnaker sign (see Appendix 1) and the thymic wave sign (see Appendix 1).

The thymus swells with crying, the Valsalva manoeuvre and after illness. It shrinks with steroids, radiation and during illness.

The *superior pericardial recess* lies behind the ascending aorta and can mimic lymphadenopathy or aortic dissection.

The *aortopulmonary window* lies between the aortic arch above and the left pulmonary artery below. It contains the ligamentum arteriosum and the recurrent laryngeal nerve. Lymphadenopathy here can cause a left recurrent laryngeal nerve palsy.

The *retrocrural space* is the lower part of the mediastinum behind the diaphragmatic crura. Here the descending aorta leaves the chest, and the azygos and hemiazygos veins are the direct continuation of the upper lumbar veins. The thoracic duct formed from the cisterna chyli also enters the chest.

Heart

The anatomy of the margins and configuration of the characteristic cardiovascular silhouette need to be understood so that abnormalities can be detected.

One-third of the heart lies to the right of the mid-line and two-thirds to the left, with the cardiac apex pointing downwards and outwards to produce the characteristic shape. In the normal adult, the transverse diameter of the cardiac silhouette is less than half the thoracic diameter.

In the frontal projection (see Fig. 2.7), the right heart border is made up entirely by the right lateral margin of the right atrium; the right heart border is outlined by the adjacent aerated medial segment of the middle lobe. The left border of the cardiovascular silhouette has four protuberances—the aortic knob, pulmonary artery, left atrial appendage and left ventricle (from top downwards). The left heart border is formed by the left ventricle margin silhouetted by the aerated lingular segments of the left upper lobe.

Fig. 2.7 Heart anatomy: frontal projection

The right heart border is formed by the right atrium (RA) with the right mediastinal border formed by the SVC.

The left ventricle (LV) forms the left heart border. The left margin of the right ventricle (RV) is about a finger's breadth in from the left heart border, corresponding to the anterior interventricular groove.

From above downwards, the heart valves are the pulmonary valve (PV), aortic valve (AV), mitral valve (MV) and tricuspid valve (TV).

Within the mediastinum, the main pulmonary artery (PA) lies to the left of the ascending aorta (AA).

The anterior margin of the heart on the lateral CXR (see Fig. 2.8) is formed by the front wall of the right ventricle; the main pulmonary artery and ascending aorta lie above.

The posterior margin of the heart is formed by the posterior margin of the left atrium.

Because of the attachment of the pericardium to the diaphragm, the heart elongates during inspiration and flattens during expiration.

Lymphatic drainage

In the secondary pulmonary nodule, lymphatic vessels are seen accompanying the veins in the interlobular septa and also accompanying the bronchoarterial bundle centrally. These lymphatic vessels converge

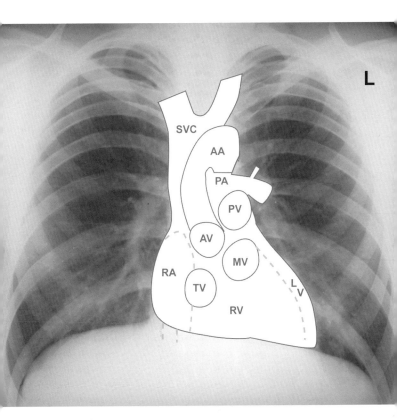

to form a deep network accompanying the blood vessels and bronchi towards the bronchopulmonary lymph nodes at the hila. There is also a superficial plexus, which drains the visceral pleura and subpleural lung, that also passes to the bronchopulmonary lymph nodes.

Flow is then via tracheobronchial and paratracheal lymph nodes into bronchomediastinal trunks, which either join the right jugular lymph trunk or thoracic duct or enter independently into the brachiocephalic veins. At their terminations they may communicate with scalene lymph nodes.

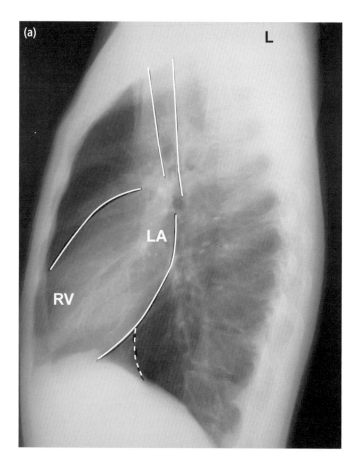

The exception to the 'homolateral' drainage of the lungs is the left lower lobe and lingula, where the flow passes from the left bronchopulmonary lymph nodes to the carinal lymph nodes and then along the right lymphatic route.

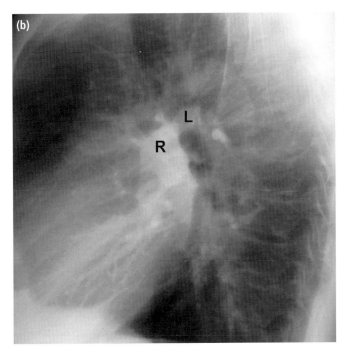

Fig. 2.8 Heart anatomy: (a) lateral view; (b) localised lateral view

(a) The cardiac margins and trachea have been highlighted. The anterior margin of the heart is the right ventricle (RV); the posterior margin is the left atrium (LA). The retrosternal and retrocardiac airspaces should have a similar radiolucency. Both hemidiaphragms are visualised and both costophrenic angles are sharp. The lower vertebral bodies are overlaid by an increasing amount of translucent lung.

(b) The trachea can be followed downwards and the lower part of the air column is the major bronchi. The rounded lucency is the left upper lobe bronchus seen end-on.

The left pulmonary artery (L) curves over the left main bronchus. The right pulmonary artery (R) is projected as a circular opacity anterior to the airway.

Bones

The density of the bones can hide the fine detail of the lungs. On a good CXR, the radiographer has positioned the patient's arm to rotate the scapulae away from being projected over the lung fields.

The lung apices do not lie higher than the posterior aspects of the first ribs but this is higher than the level of the first costal cartilages. The front of the apices, above the clavicles, are therefore exposed to possible injury (e.g. iatrogenic pneumothorax from inadvertent needle puncture).

The second costal cartilage joins the sternum at the manubriosternal junction.

Soft tissues

The thickness of the soft tissue on the chest wall varies depending on the size of the patient. In female patients, the breasts project increased density over the lower zones. In male patients and small-breasted female patients, beware of nipple shadows projected over the lower zones being misinterpreted as nodules.

Chapter 3

Chest X-ray interpretation

The best way to inspect a chest radiograph is with a good viewing box (or monitor) and in calm surroundings. An additional 'bright light' should be available for inspecting any dark areas of the film.

Novices can reduce the chance of missing an abnormality by having a directed systematic search pattern rather than a free global search. A checklist is shown in Table 3.1.

Systematic search pattern

Documentation

The film should record the patient's name, date and where it was taken. The radiographer should indicate on the film the patient's side and any change from the normal technique (i.e. anteroposterior [AP], mobile, supine, expiratory).

Technique

The film reader needs to be aware of the technique used for proper interpretation (e.g. assessment of heart size will not be valid on an AP film). Poor film centring, incorrect exposure or rotation will produce a less than ideal film and limit the diagnostic information.

Upper mediastinum

The mediastinum appears as a number of structures superimposed on one another.

Table 3.1 Checklist for scrutiny of a chest radiograph	
Frontal	**Lateral**
• Patient name and date	• Patient name and date
• Technique	• Technique
• Upper mediastinum including trachea	• Trachea
• Hila	• Hilar density and main pulmonary arteries
• Heart	• Heart and great vessels
• Diaphragm and below	• Diaphragm and below
• Lung fields: Check margins Compare zones	• Pleural fissures: Retrosternal space Retrocardiac space Posterior costophrenic angles
• Bones	• Thoracic spine, ribs
• Soft tissues	• Soft tissues
• Overall review	• Overall review
• Check for pneumothorax	
• Are there previous films for comparison?	

- The trachea should be of uniform calibre. It enters the thoracic inlet in the middle and passes slightly to the right as it passes the aortic arch. It may be displaced or compressed by a goitre or lymphadenopathy. An obstructing tracheal tumour could cause dyspnoea or a wheeze.
- The aortic knuckle is reduced in coarctation (see Fig. 3.1) and left-to-right shunts. The aortic knuckle could be widened if aneurysmal.

Look for any changes in the outline or width of the superior mediastinum that could indicate that a mass is present. The commonest cause of a widened mediastinum is ectasia or unfolding of the aortic arch and innominate artery with ageing due to the loss of elastic tissue.

Remember that the superior mediastinum, including the trachea, as well as the heart, will be shifted *towards* a collapsed lung and *away* from a large pleural effusion (see Figs 3.2, 3.3) or tension pneumothorax (see Fig. 3.4).

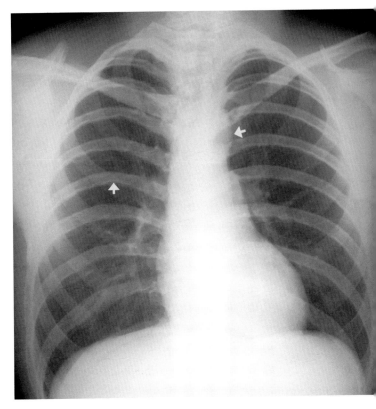

Fig. 3.1 Aortic coarctation: PA view

Coarctation of the aorta is a congenital short segment narrowing of the distal aortic arch just beyond the origin of the left subclavian artery; at or just beyond the ligamentum arteriosum.

The plain film shows the small appearing aortic knuckle. Sometimes the left paravertebral shadow is widened due to the hypertrophied left subclavian artery.

If a barium swallow was performed, the oesophagus would be identified by the dilated portions of the aorta just proximal and just distal to the coarctation.

Inferior notching of the adult fourth to eight ribs is sometimes more easily seen than the aortic abnormalities. The notching is from the pulsatile retrograde flow in the dilated intercostal arteries supplying blood to the descending aorta.

Possible associated abnormalities are congenital heart disease, including bicuspid aortic valve, intracranial berry aneurysms and Turner's syndrome (see differential diagnosis of inferior rib notching, Appendix 2).

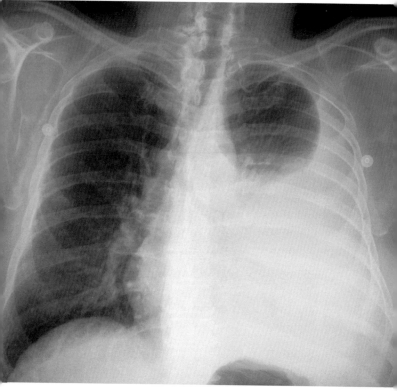

Fig. 3.2 Pleural effusion: PA view

A large, left pleural effusion is present causing a homogeneous opacity with a characteristic concave upper margin—meniscus shape. The underlying lung will be passively collapsed with more blood being delivered into the right pulmonary circulation. There is mediastinal shift to the right with the left heart border obscured. Inversion of the left hemidiaphragm has produced displacement of the gastric gas shadow.

Remember that different fluids, such as transudates or exudates, are going to have similar appearances because of their similar X-ray density. The actual cause of the effusion may need to be established from the history, other clinical or radiological findings or analysis of the aspirate itself. The common causes of a unilateral pleural effusion are infection, tumour—either primary or secondary, haemorrhage or chylothorax.

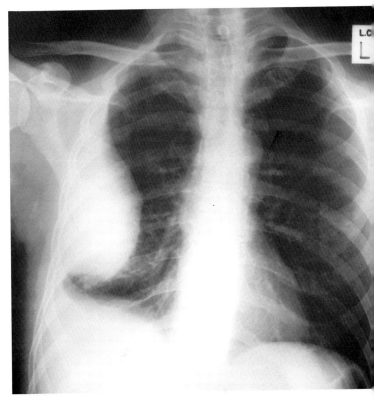

Fig. 3.3 Loculated pleural effusion: AP view

There is a large, right pleural-based opacity. Its shape indicates that it is externally loculated and by inference there are also internal loculations formed. Its upper edge is seen to taper into the pleural margin. Associated elevation of the right hemidiaphragm and blunting of the right costophrenic angle are also seen.

No rib erosion or evidence of osteomyelitis is present to suggest spread of either possible tumour or infection. The term 'empyema necissitans' is used where there is extension of the infection through the chest wall.

Confirmation that this is loculated pleural fluid could be established by ultrasound or CT scanning. (See D sign, Appendix 1.)

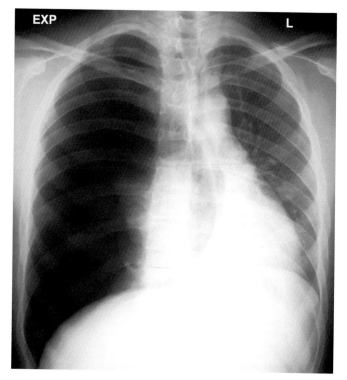

Fig. 3.4 Tension pneumothorax: PA view

Tension pneumothorax is a medical emergency. Therefore, clinical or radiological recognition is very important. Clinically, these patients are hypoxic with haemodynamic collapse.

The classic features demonstrated in this case are the shift of the trachea and mediastinum to the left, depression of the right hemidiaphragm and compression of the right lung. The markedly increased translucent right pleural space projects beyond the mid-line into the left hemithorax.

The air leak is through a tear, which behaves like a valve. The air leaks out on inspiration due to negative pleural pressure and is then under tension in the neutral and expiratory phases.

Paradoxically, the density of the collapsing lung changes very little because the blood flow diminishes in parallel.

If the underlying lung is stiff or consolidated, there can be significant tension, even if little lung collapse is present.

Drainage of a tension pneumothorax may result in an uncommon complication of re-expansion pulmonary oedema.

Hila

The left hilum will be 1–2 cm higher than the right hilum mainly because the left main pulmonary artery passes up and over the left main bronchus. The right hilum has a V-shape, with the left hilum being squarer. Even though there is a difference in the positions and shapes, the hila should have the same density. A dense hilum could be due to a lymphadenopathy or an adjacent confluent mass.

When hilar lymphadenopathy is present, it is important to distinguish between lymphadenopathy or arteriomegaly. Scrutinise the film to see if there are other sites of lymphadenopathy or whether there are prominent vessels just outside the hilum (see Fig. 3.5). The vascular causes of enlarged hila are pulmonary hypertension seen in left-to-right shunts, emphysema (see Fig. 3.6) and chronic pulmonary emboli. A hilum may appear prominent when a large acute embolus is present (Fleischner sign, see Appendix 1).

Heart

Two-thirds of the heart lie to the left of the mid-line with the bulk of the heart projected over the left lower zone. Fat pads may blunt the cardiophrenic angles. The heart borders (see Fig. 3.7) should be sharp. If not, the adjacent lung could be consolidated or collapsed (Silhouette sign, see Appendix 1). The right heart border may be absent in pectus excavatum.

Enlargement of the right atrium causes the right heart border to bulge. Marked deviation and enlargement is seen with Ebstein's anomaly.

Right ventricular enlargement produces a cardiac apex that points upwards and outwards on the frontal film (e.g. cœur en sabot shape in tetralogy of Fallot). The right ventricle forms the anterior cardiac margin and, with enlargement, more of the anterior margin bulges against the sternum.

Left atrial enlargement causes a bulge of the posterior cardiac margin. In the past this was confirmed by the lateral barium swallow view showing the indentation on the oesophagus. Nowadays, it is confirmed by echocardiography.

The left atrial appendage enlarges with left atrial enlargement and can produce the third mogul (first mogul is the aortic arch, second mogul is the pulmonary artery at the left hilum).

The left ventricle is the major cardiac chamber. As it enlarges the cardiac shadow generally enlarges and the apex points further outwards and downwards.

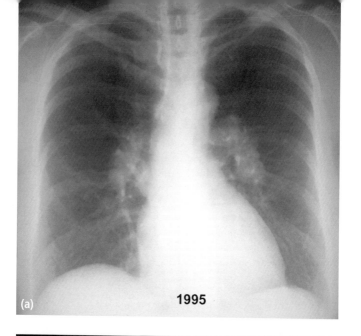

(a) 1995

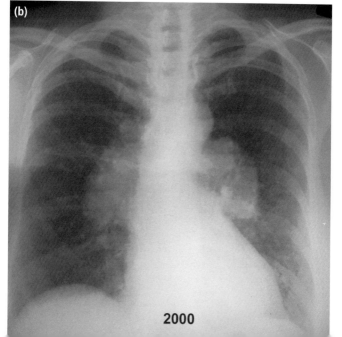

(b) 2000

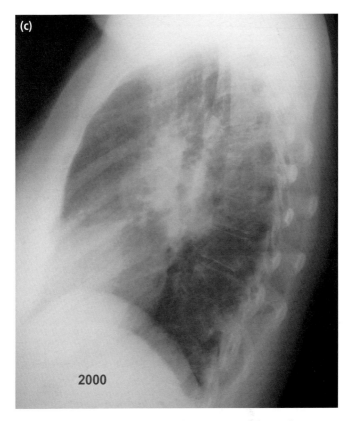

Fig. 3.5 Bilateral hilar lymphadenopathy: (a) PA view; (b) PA view; (c) lateral view

The first interpretative decision to make when enlarged hila are recognised is whether the hilar enlargement is due to lymphadenopathy or enlarged pulmonary arteries.

(a) The 1995 CXR shows a 'clear space' between the hilum and the mediastinum. This floating hilum sign (see Appendix 1) distinguishes hilar lymphadenopathy from mediastinal lymphadenopathy.

(b) By 2000, the hilar lymphadenopathy has further increased.

(c) This lateral view also shows the hilar lymphadenopathy.

Hilar symmetry is unusual in the major alternative diagnoses of lymphoma, tuberculosis and metastases. (See the differential diagnosis of hilar lymphadenopathy, Appendix 2.)

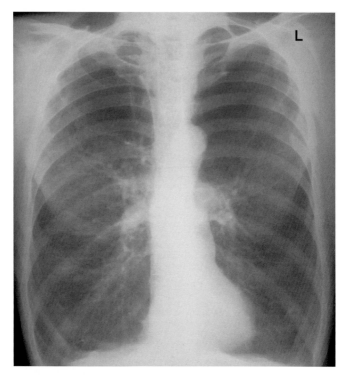

Fig. 3.6 Emphysema: PA view

Emphysema is defined as a lung disease characterised by abnormal permanent enlargement of the air spaces distal to the terminal bronchiole. There is accompanying destruction of the distal air space walls without fibrosis and also loss of the local elastic network.

This radiograph of a case of severe emphysema shows the classic features of over-inflation, oligaemia, parenchymal lung destruction and bullae formation. The resultant pulmonary hypertension is reflected in the prominence of the central pulmonary arteries. A 'hanging drop heart' may be another sign.

The lateral CXR would show an increase in the AP diameter of the chest, an increase in the retrosternal airspace and flattening of the hemidiaphragms.

Key points:
- CXR is insensitive for mild and moderate emphysema.
- CXR reliably detects severe emphysema and can be used to exclude severe disease.
- Over-inflation needs to be assessed in regard to age, body habitus.
- Other causes of chronic obstructive pulmonary disease (COPD) are chronic bronchitis, bronchiolitis obliterans, asthma.

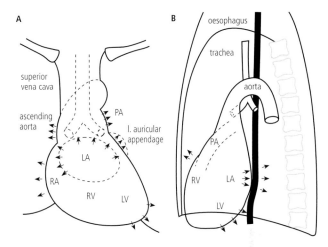

Fig. 3.7 The cardiac borders change with selective chamber enlargement
The arrows indicate the different directions with the enlargement of different chambers (RA=right atrium; RV=right ventricle; LA=left atrium; LV=left ventricle; PA=pulmonary artery). From *Clinical Radiology for Medical Students and Health Practitioners,* 2nd edn, Hare, WSC, ISBN 0 86793 007 1, Blackwell Science Asia, 1999, p. 46, reproduced with permission.

A normal-sized heart should have a transverse diameter that is less than 50% of the transthoracic diameter on a posteroanterior (PA) X-ray. Left ventricular hypertrophy does not cause recognisable cardiomegaly on the PA film. It is only in patients with heart failure and ventricular dilatation or those with pericardial effusion that the cardiothoracic ratio will exceed 50%. On AP views, the heart is further away from the film and appears larger, and hence the 50% rule cannot be used in AP X-rays.

Factors that may mimic cardiac enlargement, such as poor inspiration, abdominal distension, pectus excavatum and large fat pads, need to be excluded. If a pericardial effusion is suspected, this is best confirmed by ultrasound.

If the heart is enlarged, look for selective chamber enlargement. A double right heart border may indicate an enlarged left atrium due to mitral valve disease. The right atrium will be selectively enlarged in Ebstein's anomaly.

Calcification of the aortic and mitral valves needs to be sought within the heart shadow. A dense curved or annular calcified band around the mitral valve indicates mitral annulus calcification, which is usually not significant but can cause insufficiency if rigid.

A double density or an air–fluid level behind the heart may suggest a hiatus hernia.

Diaphragm

On the PA X-ray, the hemidiaphragms have convex, smooth upper margins. They represent the highest edge of this curved structure tangential to the X-ray beam. With good inspiration, the apex of each hemidiaphragm should reach the level of the sixth costal cartilage anteriorly and at least the tenth rib posteriorly. The right hemi-diaphragm is usually 2 cm higher than the left and has the bulk of the liver beneath it. If the diaphragmatic outline is lost, it means that there is adjacent fluid, consolidation or collapse. Pleural effusions will blunt the costophrenic angles.

In normal patients the height of the hemidiaphragm curve on both the PA and lateral view is about 2 cm. In chronic airways limitation disease the hemidiaphragms will appear flat.

Free gas under the diaphragm seen on erect views usually indicates rupture of a hollow viscus.

Lung fields

The lung fields should be equally translucent. The 'lung markings' are the blood-filled pulmonary vessels and not the bronchi. The pulmonary arteries radiate from the hila; the pulmonary veins radiate into the left atrium.

For convenience, the lung fields on the frontal view are divided into zones. The upper zones are between the lung apices and the level of the second costal cartilages. The mid-zones are between the second and fourth costal cartilage levels, and the lower zones are between the level of the fourth costal cartilage and the diaphragm. The apices lie above the clavicles; the lung bases are the lowest 2 cm.

Compare one side with the other. It is at this time that nodules, consolidation and atelectasis are usually recognised.

Consolidation means that the airspaces are filled with material which replaces the air (see Fig. 3.8). This could be an exudate,

➤

Fig. 3.8 Patterns of lobar consolidation
(a) right upper lobe; (b) middle lobe; (c) right lower lobe; (d) left upper lobe; (e) left lower lobe

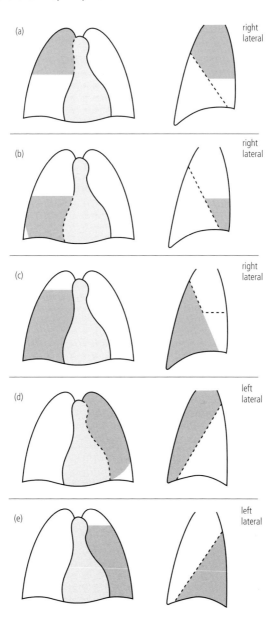

transudate, blood, protein or even tumour cells—it can sometimes be difficult to distinguish infection, oedema or infarction as a cause of an opaque lung. Bronchial obstruction by a tumour can cause distal consolidation or collapse. A collapsed lung appears opaque because the air has been lost (it is therefore wrong to call it 'collapse–consolidation') (see Figs 3.9–3.13).

An air bronchogram sign (see Appendix 1) occurs when air is seen in a bronchus because the surrounding parenchyma is opacified. This is abnormal when seen beyond the second branching of the bronchi. The horizontal fissure is visible in two-thirds of patients as a thin, opaque line at the level of the fourth costal cartilage. It passes on the PA view from the lateral aspect of the sixth rib to the right hilum. The horizontal fissure will be raised in collapse or deflationary change of the right upper lobe.

The commonest lobar collapse is that of the left lower lobe, but it is the one most easily missed. The signs are double density behind the heart, loss of outline of the medial left hemidiaphragm, and tucking-in of the left hilum.

➤

Fig. 3.9 Patterns of lobar collapse

(a) *Right upper lobe collapse.* The horizontal fissure is drawn upwards and the major fissure above the hilum is displaced anteriorly.

(b) *Right middle lobe collapse.* In both projections the horizontal fissure is drawn downwards towards the right heart border. The lateral view shows that the lower part of the major fissure is displaced forwards.

(c) *Right lower lobe collapse.* On the lateral view, the whole of the oblique fissure is displaced backwards. The major fissure is not visible on the PA view until the collapse is almost complete.

(d) *Left upper lobe collapse.* On the lateral view, the whole of the fissure is displaced upwards and anteriorly. The major fissure does not become visible on the PA projection. There is a band of translucency adjacent to the aortic arch (Luftsichel sign, see Appendix 1). Otherwise, loss of translucency is seen in the left upper and mid-zones. Note that there is a major difference in the pattern of collapse between the right upper and left upper lobes.

(e) *Left lower lobe collapse.* The lateral view shows that the major fissure is displaced posteriorly as in collapse of the right lower lobe. The collapsed lobe is seen as a triangular density projected behind the cardiac shadow. Compensatory over-inflation of the left upper lobe occurs with splaying of its pulmonary vessels.

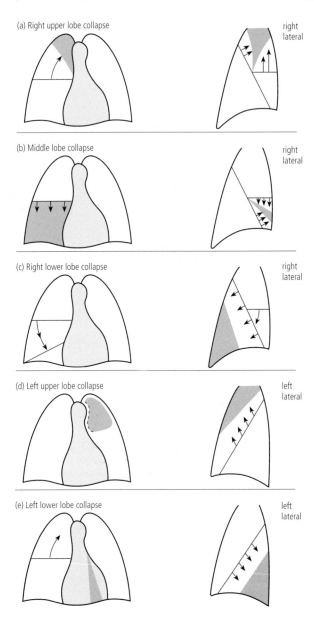

(a) Right upper lobe collapse — right lateral

(b) Middle lobe collapse — right lateral

(c) Right lower lobe collapse — right lateral

(d) Left upper lobe collapse — left lateral

(e) Left lower lobe collapse — left lateral

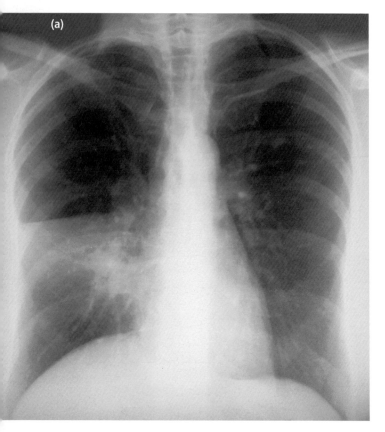

Fig. 3.10 Middle lobe collapse: (a) PA view; (b) lateral view

The airless middle lobe lies against the right heart border and has produced loss of the cardiac outline, the so-called silhouette sign (see Appendix 1). Because the middle lobe has a small volume, no recognisable changes are seen in the right hilum or right pulmonary vessels.

On the lateral radiograph there is a wedge-shaped opacity from the horizontal fissure displaced inferiorly and the lower half of the oblique fissure displaced superiorly.

CT scanning or bronchoscopy will be necessary to ascertain whether it is an obstructive atelectasis from a central tumour.

The right middle lobe syndrome is a pattern of recurrent or chronic atelectasis due to extrinsic lymph node compression of the lobar bronchus and poor collateral ventilation.

(b)

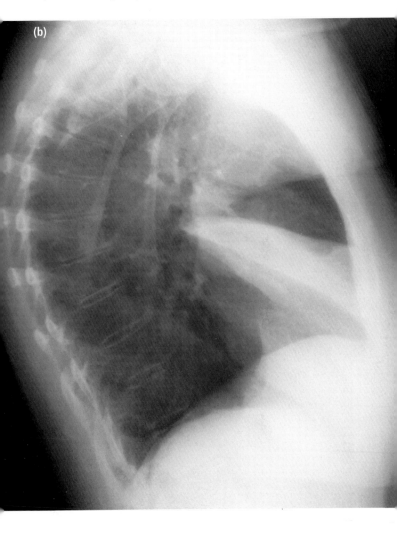

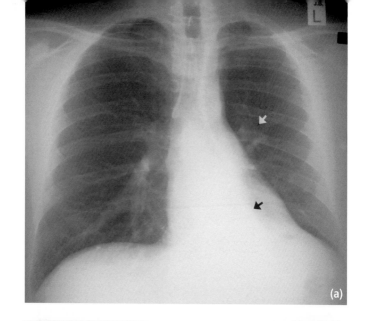

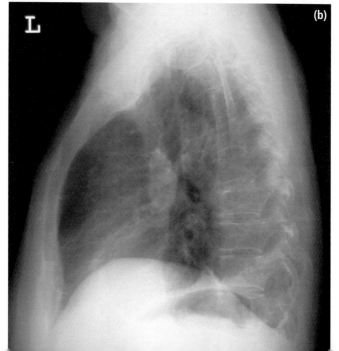

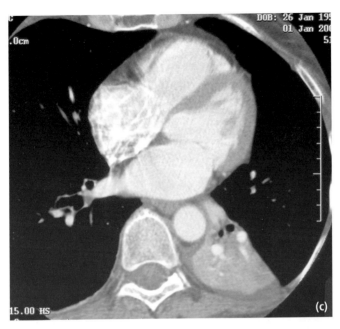

Fig. 3.11 Left lower lobe collapse: (a) PA view; (b) lateral view; (c) CT scan
Left lower lobe collapse is the most common lobar collapse and the most difficult to recognise.

The lobe collapses posteromedially against the posterior mediastinum and spine. On the PA view it appears as a triangular opacity behind the heart and adjacent to the spine (black arrow).

Other signs are the inferior displacement of the left hilum (white arrow), leftward shift of the heart, elevation and poor visualisation of the left hemidiaphragm, and compensatory hyperinflation of the left upper lobe. Also there is flattening of the left cardiac border—the flat waist sign (see Appendix 1).

Bronchoscopy is indicated to ascertain the cause for the collapse. Obstructive atelectasis could be due to an endobronchial tumour or an extrinsic mass. In postoperative and ill patients, a mucous plug may be the cause and will need removal.

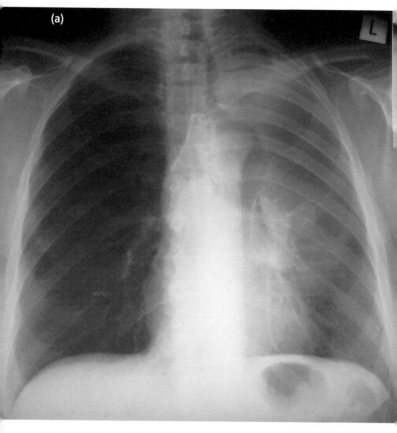

Fig. 3.12 Left upper lobe collapse: (a) PA view; (b) lateral view; (c) CT scan
On the frontal film, there is decreased translucency in the left upper and mid-zones, loss of the left heart border silhouette, leftward superior mediastinal shift, a high position of the left hemidiaphragm, and the luftsichel sign (see Appendix 1). In addition, there is a left hilar mass indicating that the collapse is due to tumour obstruction of the left upper lobe bronchus (also well shown on the CT scan).

The characteristic forward deviation of the major fissure is seen on the lateral view, with the collapsed lobe seen as a triangular opacity. On the CT scan, note the aerated lung adjacent to the upper part of the descending aorta to help explain the luftsichel sign (see Appendix 1). Herniation of right lung is also seen across the mid-line, anterior to the ascending aorta, on the CT scan and the lateral view.

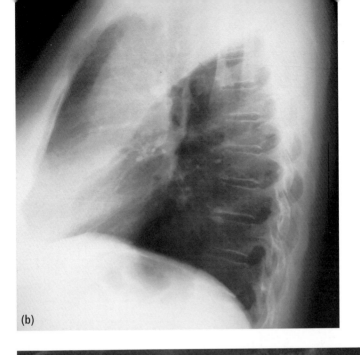

(b)

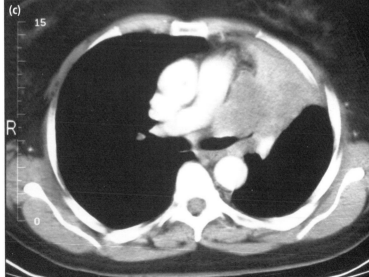

(c)

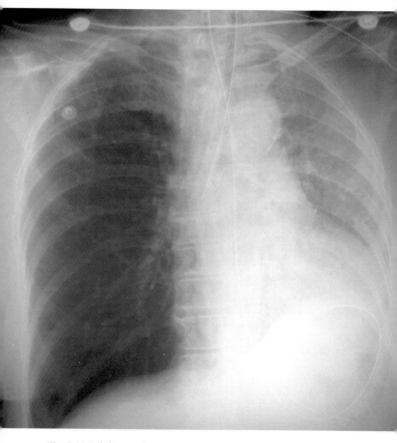

Fig. 3.13 Left lung collapse: PA view

Inadvertent intubation of the right main bronchus has restricted the aeration of the left lung causing incomplete collapse.

The left lung is small with increased opacification, leftward shift of the mediastinum and elevation of the left hemidiaphragm.

The right main bronchus is more vertical in orientation and therefore more likely to be selectively intubated. Sometimes intubation of the right main bronchus can cause collapse of the right upper lobe as well.

If the heart is enlarged, check for further signs of heart failure and oedema. Possible findings range from pulmonary venous congestion, interstitial oedema to alveolar oedema with pleural effusion.

Scrutinise the edges of the lung fields for any pleural abnormalities—effusion, plaque or calcification. When fluid accumulates in the pleural space it appears opaque and causes passive atelectasis of the adjacent lung. The pleural fluid could be a transudate, exudate, blood or chyle. If the effusion is free, it will show a characteristic meniscus sign on X-rays taken with the patient standing. Remember that some posterior basal lung lies below the apex of the hemidiaphragm on the PA film.

Bones

A quick perusal of the ribs, clavicles, scapulas and lower cervical spine should follow. The ribs and intercostal spaces should have symmetrical widths and shape. If there is a specific concern about rib fractures, then more attention is necessary. Subtle, undisplaced fractures of the lateral ribs are better observed with the film rotated on the viewing box so that the observer can scan the lateral rib edges horizontally.

Inferior rib notching occurs with coarctation of the aorta but there are other causes.

Costal cartilage calcification in elderly patients occurs at the margins in men and centrally in women. Note if a cervical rib is present. Note that scoliosis of the thoracic spine frequently accounts for mediastinal distortions. Look at the paraspinal lines behind the heart and mediastinum. They can be displaced in trauma, infectious spondylodiscitis and posterior mediastinal masses.

Soft tissues

In women, the soft tissues of the breast appear as shadows. Women with large breasts will have increased density over the lower zones. Alternatively, if there has been a mastectomy, the lower zone lung on that side will appear more transradient. Further, radiation fibrosis may explain any upper-zone scarring (see Fig. 3.14).

Soft tissues include those seen below the diaphragm. A CXR may show such abnormalities as calcified hydatid cysts in the liver and splenomegaly (which displaces the gastric air bubble under the left hemidiaphragm). If barium is seen in the bowel, this may be a clue that the patient has another problem which has already been investigated.

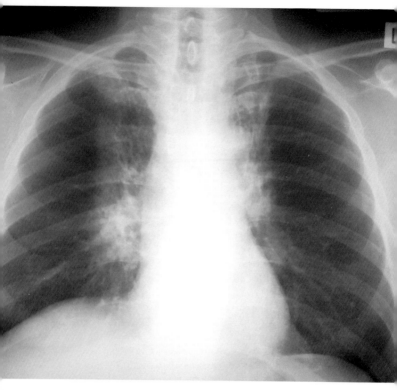

Fig. 3.14 Radiation fibrosis: PA view

Radiation therapy may injure the exposed lung firstly by an acute phase of radiation pneumonitis and then by fibrosis. The sharp lateral borders, as seen in this case, correspond to the radiation ports rather than any anatomical boundary.

The fibrosis is shown as coarse, linear stranding. With further progressive fibrosis, volume loss will occur with elevation of the hila.

Review

A second look at the lung fields partially obscured by the ribs, clavicles and heart is the next step. Most missed lesions lie in the apices, behind the medial ends of the clavicles or behind the left side of the heart. Because the apices are a common site for post-primary tuberculosis, a lordotic AP view may be needed. This will project the clavicles above the apices for better visualisation.

Table 3.2 shows the common pitfalls in interpreting CXRs and Table 3.3 shows false negative causes of CXR interpretation.

Table 3.2 Common pitfalls in interpreting chest X-rays
1. Wrong patient/wrong film/wrong date.
2. Not recognising a post-mastectomy chest wall in a female patient.
3. Mistaking costal cartilage calcification in elderly patients for intrathoracic disease.
4. The lung fields may appear plethoric with crowded markings, the mediastinum widened and the diaphragm elevated in expiratory or supine chest films.
5. Not recognising skinfolds as a cause of an opacity or margin, or confusing a skinfold with a pneumothorax.
6. Incorrect diagnosis of cardiomegaly on a mobile or anteroposterior film.
7. Confusing a nipple shadow for a pulmonary nodule (the nipple shadows can be distinguished from other rounded opacities in the lower zones by skin markers).
8. Not recognising that the loss of elastic tissue in the aorta and main branches results in an 'unfolded aorta', which occurs with age and may mimic paratracheal masses.
9. Not recognising that pectus excavatum may compress the heart, which then appears as 'cardiomegaly'.
10. Not recognising spurious 'hilar' lesions where the hilar margins are visible through the opacity (e.g. an apical lesion in the lower lobe projected over the hilum on the frontal film)—see hilum overlay sign (Appendix 1).
11. Not knowing that extrapleural lipomatosis in obese patients can simulate pleural thickening.

Table 3.3 Reasons for false negative chest X-ray interpretation

- Faulty visual search
- Satisfaction of search effect (search is terminated after discovery of an abnormality)
- Faulty pattern recognition
- Faulty decision making

Pneumothorax

In any ordered scrutiny of the CXR film it is worthwhile checking for a small pneumothorax, especially in hospitalised patients. The pneumothorax may be hard to see because the low density of the inflated lung periphery and the free pleural gas are similar (see Figs 3.15, 3.16). Beware of missing a pneumothorax on an over-penetrated CXR in which the lung fields are dark.

If a pneumothorax is large, it could be under tension, which is life-threatening for the patient. The signs are:
- the mediastinum is shifted away
- the diaphragm is displaced downwards and the lung is collapsed.

These signs are even more dramatic on the expiratory film.

──▶

Fig. 3.15 Pneumothorax: PA view
The pleural space is normally a potential space with only a small amount of lubricating pleural fluid present. *Pneumothorax* literally means free air in the pleural space between the parietal pleura and the visceral pleura. It can be difficult to distinguish density differences between the free air and the peripheral lung where no vascular shadows are present. The pneumothorax is easier to see on expiratory films as the size of the pneumothorax remains constant and the deflated lung becomes denser.

The visceral pleural line (arrowed) is thin.

Even a small pneumothorax is important to identify as it may rapidly increase in size in patients being artificially ventilated. For practical purposes, a pneumothorax can be reported as small, medium or large. Occasionally, clinicians may want an estimation of the pneumothorax size (see Collins CD et al. Quantification of pneumothorax size on chest radiographs using interpleural distances. *AJR* 1995;165:1127).

In this case, the 1 cm rim of pneumothorax is occupying about 15–20%. However, the patient's clinical status is more important than the exact percentage of collapse. (See differential diagnosis of pneumothorax, Appendix 2.)

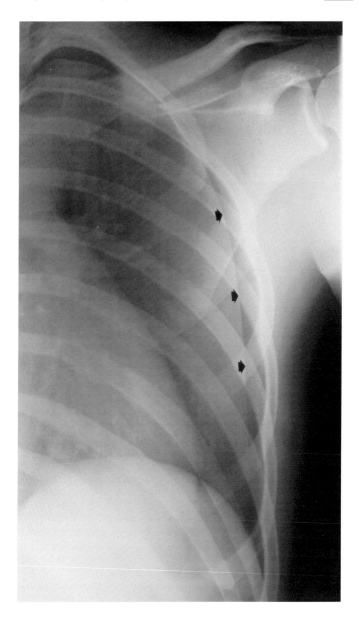

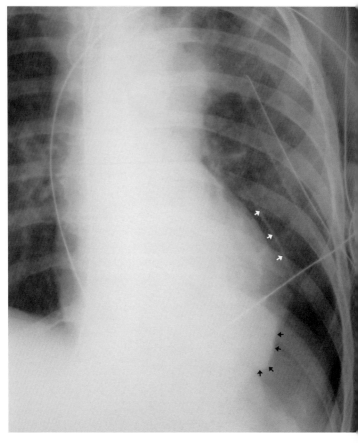

Fig. 3.16 Basal supine pneumothorax: AP view

Despite the presence of a chest tube, a left pneumothorax is present in this supine patient. It has risen to the highest part of the hemithorax in the anterior costophrenic angle. These basal supine pneumothoraces can be difficult to identify because the visceral pleural edge may not be separated from the apex or lateral chest wall. The visceral pleural edge is separated from the left cardiac margin (white arrows). The free air sharpens the cardiac outline (black arrows).

In this case there is also a band of subcutaneous emphysema lying on the outer edges of the ribs.

See the anterior sulcus sign (Appendix 1), deep sulcus sign (Appendix 1) and double diaphragm sign (Appendix 1).

Considerations in the young

Broadly speaking, CXRs in infants and children are indicated when there is a need to check the airways and lung fields, and to check for any gross cardiac anomalies. Ideally, the radiograph (usually an AP view for convenience) should be taken when patients are still and during full inspiration, although an expiratory X-ray may be helpful if there is concern about a foreign body and signs of air-trapping are recognised.

In young children the lung fields are relatively small and the diaphragm high. Congenital abnormalities that can be detected include diaphragmatic hernia, lung hypoplasia and lobar emphysema. The radiographic signs of asthma are more common in children than adults and include hyperinflation and bronchial wall thickening. The mediastinum is prominent because of the thymus. The thymic shadow is relatively large in the first three years and then diminishes (the thymic shadow should not be confused with lung consolidation—see Sail sign, Appendix 1).

Considerations in the elderly

Age-related changes should be noted in the elderly (see Table 3.4). For example, in the spine, there is increasing thoracic kyphosis with

Table 3.4	Normal signs of advanced age

- Calcified costal cartilages
- Calcified trachea and main bronchi
- Degenerative spinal disc disease with disc space narrowing and osteophytes
- Demineralisation of the thoracic spine and increased kyphosis
- Aortic wall calcification
- Loss of elastic tissue causing 'unfolding' of the aorta and arch branches. The ascending aorta projects further to the right than the superior vena cava (SVC) so that its convex border forms the right mediastinal outline
- With unfolding and ectasia of the aortic arch, the trachea deviates more to the right as it descends
- Tortuous descending aorta
- Apical lung scarring
- The lower flatter hemidiaphragms and the altered thoracic shape produce an appearance of 'senile emphysema'

osteoporosis and osteophytic lipping with degenerative change. Osteophytes can also be seen in the glenohumeral and acromio-clavicular joints. Calcification is common in the costal cartilages, trachea and bronchi. Note that the aorta 'unfolds' with loss of elastic tissue, as it is fixed at the aortic valve and the diaphragm hiatus. The ascending aorta bulges the right border of the upper mediastinum and the descending aorta bulges to the left. Generalised tissue wasting occurs. The loss of lung volume is accompanied by collapse of the chest wall inwards. This increases the cardiothoracic ratio to more than 50%, even when the heart itself is smaller (see Fig. 3.17). Further, loss of peripheral lung vessels leads to increased pulmonary resistance, pulmonary hypertension and prominence of the pulmonary trunks (hila).

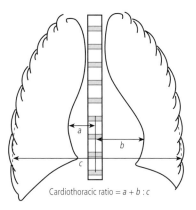

Cardiothoracic ratio = $a + b : c$

Fig. 3.17 Estimation of the cardiothoracic ratio

Lateral chest X-ray

The lateral view is necessary to provide further information when an abnormality is seen on the PA film. Usually the left lateral view is the routine. As with the PA view, this film is viewed from the 'film' side of the patient, so that for the left lateral view the film is placed with the sternum on the examiner's left. There should be a sequence of search or a mental checklist so that scrutiny is complete.

- The name and date needed to be checked first so that the study corresponds to the PA view.
- Apart from satisfactory film exposure, a good technique is that the arms are elevated so that they do not hide lung detail. Check whether the ribs overlap and that there is no rotation.
- The trachea should be followed downwards from the neck to a rounded translucency—this does not correspond to the true anatomical carina. This rounded translucency represents the main bronchi.
- Check the density of the hilar shadows. The right pulmonary artery should lie anterior to the 'carina' with the left pulmonary artery lying above and then posterior to the 'carina'. Because the two hilar shadows are superimposed, it is difficult to distinguish the features of one from the other.
- The heart shadow lies anteroinferiorly in the chest with the ascending aorta arising superiorly and joining the aortic arch. More of the descending aorta becomes visible on the lateral film as the patient ages, loses elastic tissue or the descending aorta bulges against the lung.
- If there is any exaggerated bulge of the posterior cardiac margin, consider if left atrial dilatation is present.
- Unusual densities projected over the anterior cardiophrenic angle are most likely pericardial fat pads.
- Check for any valvular or pericardial calcifications.
- Portions of lung fields need to be assessed individually. Remember that the lateral view shows superimposition of the two lungs and therefore the vascular pattern is less informative. The retrosternal and retrocardiac air spaces should have a similar 'blackness' or translucency. The increasing amount of lung over the spine from above downwards should be blacker. If not, this suggests dense lung or fluid is projected over the spine (see Vertebral fade-off sign, Appendix 1).
- Are the pleural fissures visible?
- The diaphragm should be examined at the same time as the lung bases. Check that the costophrenic angles are sharp and not blunted by the first signs of an effusion.
- The hemidiaphragms can be traced back posteriorly to the ribs (see Big rib sign, Appendix 1). If a unilateral pleural effusion is present, only one hemidiaphragm may be visible.
- It depends on the centring whether one hemidiaphragm is projected higher than the other. If the gastric air bubble is visible, the

left hemidiaphragm should lie just above it. The hemidiaphragms may be flattened in chronic airways limitation (CAL).

- As with the PA film, check the soft tissues and bones. The thoracic spine and discs should be well visualised. Take care that the scapulae are not mistaken for lung opacities.

Another method of lateral CXR search is the ABC system—A for airways, B for bones, C for cardiac, D for diaphragm, E for effusions, F for fissures, G for gastric gas, H for hila.

Limitations of chest radiography

Chest X-rays are frequently normal in *pulmonary embolism without infarction*. If the patient is dyspnoeic and the chest radiograph is normal, always raise the possibility of pulmonary embolism in the report. Figley et al. have said 'The principal evidence of embolism on the chest roentgenogram is often the paucity of abnormalities for a patient in such dire straits'. However, a CXR is necessary to exclude other causes for symptoms of chest pain, dyspnoea or haemoptysis, for example: *small lung cancers* may be inconspicuous.

In *asthma*, the CXR may be normal or show hyperinflation, but the degree of hyperinflation correlates poorly with the severity and reversibility of the asthma attack. In *emphysema*, the CXR can show gross morphological change such as bullae, increased lung translucency and flattened hemidiaphragms, but these signs are not always present and physiological information must be gained from lung function tests and blood gas analyses. *Inflammatory changes of the bronchi* are not visible unless they produce secondary changes in the lungs or if they cause bronchial wall thickening. Hence, *bronchiectasis* is seen only when the changes have become marked. *Dry pleurisy and even small effusions* are not visible. The lateral costophrenic angles will not become blunted on a frontal or PA radiograph until 100 mL of pleural fluid has collected—the first place an effusion becomes visible is at the posterior costophrenic angles on the lateral X-ray, where 50 mL of pleural fluid needs to accumulate before it becomes visible.

Similarly, *myocardial infarction* shows no specific radiographic signs, and the purpose of the CXR is to determine the degree of pulmonary oedema and exclude other causes of chest pain.

Moderate mediastinal lymph node enlargement and other *mediastinal abnormalities* can be hidden in the uniform mediastinal density unless there is an alteration in the mediastinal contour.

The diagnostic information obtained from AP films, either erect or supine, is less than from PA films. AP films are technically more difficult for the radiographer, leading to poor patient positioning and centring, with longer exposure times required. Fine detail of the lungs and the amount of lung visualised are reduced and cardiac size cannot be assessed. Upper lobe blood diversion cannot be ascertained on supine films. These AP films are performed for bed-ridden patients to check line and tube placement, pneumothorax, lung collapse, lung consolidation and so on.

Tables 3.5 and 3.6 show structures that mimic chest abnormalities on CXR and computed tomography (CT).

Table 3.5 **Chest X-ray mimics**

Mimicked pathology	Structure
Pneumothorax	Skin fold, rib companion shadow, apical bulla, monitoring line
Pulmonary nodule	Skin mole, nipple, electrocardiogram pad, pleural plaque, sclerotic bone lesion (e.g. bone island), healing rib fracture, spinal osteophyte
Apical mass/opacity	Hair locks, first rib costochondral calcification
Lung tumour/pneumonia	Breast prosthesis, scapula, rib fusion, pseudotumour
Right upper lobe consolidation	Infant thymus (sail sign)
Middle lobe collapse	Pectus excavatum
Lung cavity	Loculated hydropneumothorax, ulcerating breast carcinoma
Mediastinal mass	Pericardial fat pad, unfolded innominate artery, right-sided aortic arch, double aortic arch, aortic coarctation, aortic pseudocoarctation, large vertebral osteophyte, consolidated azygos lobe
Cardiomegaly	Pectus excavatum, large cardiophrenic fat pads
Diaphragmatic mass	Diaphragmatic eventration
Raised hemidiaphragm	Subpulmonary effusion
Subcutaneous emphysema	Long hair braids
Pleural thickening	Extrapleural fat in an obese patient
Pneumoperitoneum	Interposition of colon above the liver (Chilaiditi syndrome)

Table 3.6 **Computed tomography mimics**

Mimicked pathology	Structure
Pulmonary embolus	Right hilar lymphatic sump of Borrie
Aortic dissection	Superior pericardial recess
Lymphadenopathy	Superior pericardial recess, aortopulmonary window

Chapter 4

Common lung pathologies

The common lung pathologies are:
- pneumonia, including tuberculosis (TB) infection
- pulmonary oedema (see Chapter 5)
- embolism
- tumour
- collapse
- haemorrhage
- emphysema
- occupational lung disease
- chronic diffuse infiltrative lung disease.

Pneumonia

Pneumonia means inflammation of the lungs. It is visualised on the radiograph as either alveolar or interstitial shadowing. Alveolar shadowing or airspace filling shows as consolidation, in this case due to an exudate. The signs of consolidation are the increased density itself, the air bronchogram sign (see Appendix 1) and the silhouette sign (see Appendix 1). Interstitial shadowing is characteristic of viral and *Pneumocystis carinii* pneumonias and shows as increased interstitial markings.

Primary pneumonia occurs in an otherwise normal lung, whereas secondary pneumonia occurs beyond bronchial occlusion, from aspiration, or in a pre-existing abnormality. The bronchial obstruction could be due to a bronchial tumour or inhaled foreign body. Aspiration may be from oropharyngeal or gastric contents, sinusitis or extrogenous fluid.

The three major aspiration syndromes are bacterial pneumonia, chemical pneumonitis and obstructive atelectasis. The aspiration of oropharyngeal flora leads to pneumonia in the gravity-dependent portions of the lungs. Aspiration of gastric juice (Mendelson's syndrome) results in acute lung injury. Aspiration of large particles can lead to obstructive atelectasis.

Acute pulmonary infection may be caused by a variety of organisms. Bacterial, mycobacterial, fungal, viral and parasitic pneumonias can all produce focal or diffuse airspace opacities on chest radiography or an interstitial pattern.

The six main radiological patterns are:

1. *Bronchopneumonia*: This starts in the airways and spreads to the peribronchial alveoli with multifocal areas of consolidation. These patchy, inhomogeneous shadows can coalesce. The bronchopneumonia pattern is commonly observed with staphylococcal infection.

2. *Lobar pneumonia*: In this case, the inflammatory changes are confined to a lobe (see Fig. 4.1). Classically, it occurs with *Streptococcus pneumoniae* but also with *Klebsiella*, primary TB and *Staphylococcus*. *Klebsiella* pneumonia can produce the bulging fissure sign (see Appendix 1) due to the associated oedema.

3. *Rounded pneumonia*: This can occur with staphylococcal infection in children and in fungal infection (e.g. aspergilloma and toruloma).

4. *Interstitial pattern*: This occurs with viral pneumonias and *Pneumocystis carinii* and occasionally with *Mycoplasma* infections.

---▶

Fig. 4.1 Right upper lobe consolidation: (a) PA view; (b) lateral view
Increased opacity is seen in the shape of the right upper lobe. The slight elevation of the horizontal fissure indicates that a degree of collapse is also present. This slight collapse would explain the rightward deviation of the trachea.

If this consolidation was more dense, the air bronchogram sign (see Appendix 1) might be visible with more loss of the mediastinal silhouette.

The commonest cause of a lobar pneumonia is *Streptococcus pneumoniae*.

If the consolidation fails to clear, an endobronchial mass causing a post-obstructive pneumonia needs to be considered (see differential diagnosis of lobar pneumonia, Appendix 2).

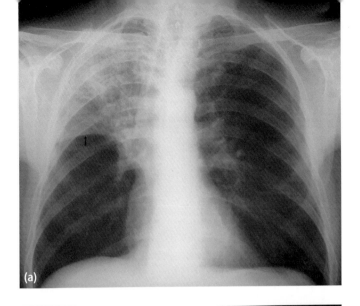

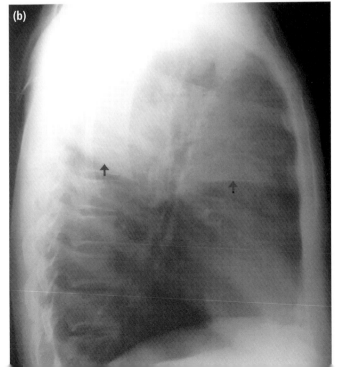

5. *Cavitatory pneumonia*: This implies that necrosis has occurred with drainage into the bronchial tree. Acute cavitation is seen with *Staphylococcus* and anaerobic bacteria. Chronic cavitation occurs with TB, histoplasmosis and coccidiomycosis (see Fig. 4.2).
6. *Miliary pneumonia* (see Fig. 4.3).

Another classification of pneumonia is based on the clinical situation in which the infection occurs:
- community-acquired pneumonia
- nosocomial pneumonia
- aspiration pneumonia
- pneumonia in the immunocompromised host.

Types of pneumonia
- In nearly half the patients, the aetiological agent is not identified.
- Streptococcal pneumonia is the commonest cause of bacterial pneumonia. The classic manifestation is a lobar pneumonia.
- Staphylococcal pneumonia is the most frequent cause of bronchopneumonia and is the usual secondary invader after viral influenza infection. It is an important cause of nosocomial infections and is a complication of infected intravenous catheters.
- Atypical pneumonia is a subset of pneumonias which do not have the typical symptoms. The patients have a non-productive cough and extrapulmonary manifestations, such as headache, myalgia and diarrhoea. Included as causes in this group of pneumonias are *Mycoplasma*, *Legionella* and *Chlamydia*. More recently the severe acute respiratory syndrome (SARS) coronavirus has caused epidemics of atypical pneumonia.
- *Mycoplasma* pneumonia usually shows as a diffuse interstitial fine reticulonodular pattern or patchy consolidation.
- Legionnaire's disease (*Legionella* pneumonia) is usually a cause of local epidemics from infected air-conditioning systems.

Fig. 4.2 Tuberculous cavity: (a) PA view; (b) lordotic view
There is a cavitating lung lesion in the right upper lobe which is partially hidden by the overlying bones on the standard PA view. The lordotic view provides a better demonstration (see differential diagnosis of cavitating lung lesion, Appendix 2).

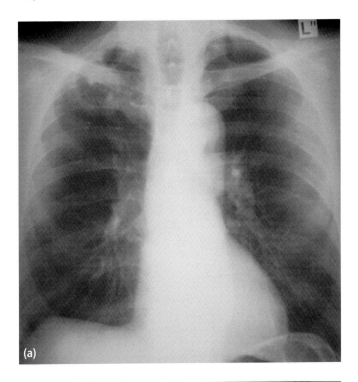

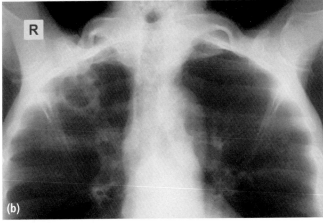

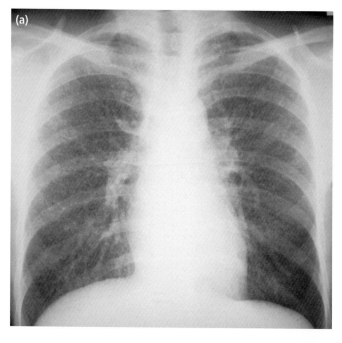

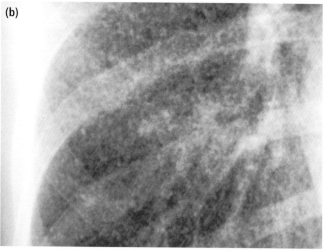

Fig. 4.3 Miliary tuberculosis: (a) PA view; (b) magnified view
The widespread multiple 1–2 mm nodules are so-called because of their resemblance of millet seeds. They are uniform in size and distribution. Massive haematogenous spread results in multiple mycobacterial foci caught in capillary sieves of the interstitium. This miliary disease may take up to six weeks to become apparent on chest radiographs, although CT may allow earlier detection of very small nodules.

Miliary tuberculosis usually occurs as a progression of primary tuberculosis but can also be a serious complication of reactivation tuberculosis. Miliary TB does *not* leave residual calcifications (see differential diagnosis of miliary nodules, Appendix 2).

- Respiratory syncytial virus (RSV) is the most common viral pneumonia in children whereas influenza is the most common in adults. The main viruses causing viral pneumonia in immuno-compromised patients are cytomegalovirus, varicella zoster and herpes.
- *Pneumocystis carinii* pneumonia is a complicating illness in acquired immunodeficiency syndrome (AIDS) or immuno-suppressed patients, including transplant patients and those on long-term steroid therapy. *Pneumocystis* is named from its cystic structure rather than the pneumatocoeles it can produce. The usual presentation shows a chest radiograph with fine symmetrical reticular opacification.
- SARS is caused by a coronavirus. The chest radiograph may show ground-glass opacity or consolidation. If the CXR is normal, then high-resolution computed tomography (HRCT) is necessary. Cavitation, calcification, lymphadenopathy and pleural effusion are not features of this disease.
- Inhalational anthrax causes a haemorrhagic pneumonia with hilar and mediastinal lymphadenopathy.
- Crytogenic-organising pneumonia is a chronic focal process of consolidation that is treated with steroids.
- Chronic eosinophilic pneumonia produces the symptoms of dyspnoea, fever, chills, night sweats and weight loss. Blood eosinophilia, peripheral consolidation and dramatic response to corticosteroid treatment are the hallmarks of diagnosis. 'Reverse butterfly' appearance on CXR.
- Lipoid pneumonia occurs usually in elderly patients and results from oil aspiration. It is not an infective pneumonia.

- Toruloma is a mass-like infection of the fungus *Crytococcus neoformans*. It can mimic a lung carcinoma.
- Nosocomial pneumonia is a general term for hospital-acquired pneumonia.
- Hydrocarbon pneumonia follows aspiration of kerosene or other hydrocarbons. It produces pulmonary oedema and lower zone opacities.

Tuberculosis

Tuberculosis is due to infection by *Mycobacterium tuberculosis*, usually in the respiratory tract.

Primary TB is usually asymptomatic, with inhalation of airborne droplets causing a focal area of consolidation with lymphadenopathy in the hilum. Lymphadenopathy may also be present in the contiguous nodes. The combination of the focal pulmonary lesion (Ghon lesion) and the lymphadenopathy is the primary Rathke complex. The enlarged lymph nodes can cause bronchial compression and obstructive atelectasis. The Ghon lesion usually heals into a focus of calcification but can persist as a tuberculoma.

A number of factors can predispose to reactivation, including malnutrition, diabetes mellitus, alcoholism, ageing, drug-induced immunosuppression, disease-induced immunosuppression and AIDS. This post-primary or reactivation TB is common in the apical and posterior segments of the upper lobes and the apical segments of the lower lobes. These segments are characterised by a high ventilation/perfusion (V/Q) ratio and relatively high Po_2 levels. A chronic patchy area of consolidation with cavitation occurs (see Fig. 4.2). Hilar and mediastinal lymphadenopathy are not a feature in immunocompetent patients.

Other patterns of reactivation include lobar pneumonia, diffuse bronchopneumonia, endobronchial TB and tuberculous pleuritis. Miliary TB is due to haematogenous dissemination and can complicate both primary and reactivation disease (see Fig. 4.3).

The healing of the pulmonary lesions is manifest by reduction in the area of consolidation, decrease in cavity size, fibrosis and calcification.

Pulmonary complications include bronchiectasis, pneumothorax, bronchopleural fistula, bronchial stenosis and broncholiths. Pleural complications are empyema and calcific fibrothorax (see Fig. 4.4).

The TB may extend to extrathoracic sites, such as the intestine, kidneys, spine and central nervous system.

The type of pulmonary TB in AIDS patients depends on the patient's CD4 lymphocyte count. If the CD4 count is below 200/µL, the pattern resembles primary TB, but if it is above 200/µL, it is more like reactivation TB.

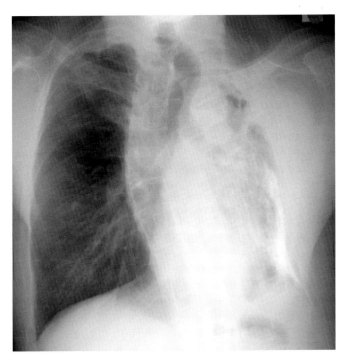

Fig. 4.4 Tuberculous calcific fibrothorax: PA view

There is gross destruction of the left lung by previous TB producing marked fibrosis. The fibrosis has shrunk the lung and caused mediastinal shift. This presumably has occurred before adult life, with a developmental scoliosis and small left hemithorax. Only a small amount of aerated left lung is present. Follow-up films or comparison with earlier films would be necessary to exclude ongoing disease.

Marked generalised pleural thickening is present with pleural calcification seen over the lower zone.

The right lung shows pleural thickening and scarring at the apex; a calcified focus is seen in the right mid-zone.

Pulmonary embolism

Pulmonary thromboembolism is a common life-threatening condition that is very difficult to diagnose solely on clinical signs and symptoms.

The chest radiograph is abnormal in most cases of pulmonary embolism (PE) but the findings are non-specific, like the clinical signs and symptoms. The non-specific findings that could be present are pleural effusion, atelectasis, parenchymal opacification and elevation of the hemidiaphragm. The classic findings of Hampton's hump sign (see Appendix 1), Westermark's sign (see Appendix 1) and Fleischner sign (see Appendix 1) are only rarely seen.

Alternatively, a normal appearing CXR in a patient with severe dyspnoea and hypoxaemia strongly suggests PE if bronchospasm and shunting have been excluded.

Since chest radiography cannot prove or exclude PE conclusively, the radiological work-up of PE requires V/Q isotope scanning, computed tomographic pulmonary angiography (CTPA) and Doppler ultrasound of the legs. The CXR is done routinely with an electrocardiogram (ECG) to identify other diagnoses. In difficult cases, pulmonary angiography may be required. However the new gold standard test may prove to be multichannel spiral computed tomography (multislice CT) after further clinical trials.

Tumour

Thoracic neoplasms can occur in the airways, lungs, mediastinum, pleura or chest wall.

A solitary pulmonary nodule is a well-circumscribed parenchymal mass 3 cm or less in diameter (see Fig. 4.5). There are a number of different diagnostic possibilities. If calcification is present within the nodule, it is most likely either a tuberculous granuloma or a hamartoma. Calcification is a good sign to exclude malignancy. Further work-up with CT scanning is required to see if it contains fat or if it has appearances suggesting infarction or pneumonia. Other forms of work-up include CT densitometry, serial CT scans with volumetric analysis and positron emission tomography (PET) with fluorodeoxy-glucose (FDG). If the nodule cannot be proven to be benign, it must be biopsied or excised.

Malignant primary tumours are divided histologically into small cell and non-small cell carcinomas. Small cell lung cancer behaves as a systemic disease and is usually disseminated at the time of diagnosis. Non-small cell lung cancer may be isolated and appropriately treated by surgical resection. Therefore, the tumour–node–metastasis (TNM) grading system is used to facilitate decision making.

The TNM grading is a system of grading of the primary tumour, regional lymph nodes and distant metastases. The International Staging System for non-small cell carcinoma further grades the tumour in terms of prognosis.

The critical division is between stages IIIA and IIIB: stage IIIA is extensive but resectable disease whereas stage IIIB is irresectable disease.

Even though chest radiography and CT scanning provide important information, other tests, such as bronchoscopy, PET scanning and mediastinoscopy, are useful in preoperative evaluation. However, the actual findings at thoracotomy will influence the surgeon's decision making.

Diffuse pulmonary haemorrhage

Diffuse pulmonary haemorrhage occurs when there is widespread haemorrhage from the lung microvasculature into the alveolar spaces. It can occur with conditions associated with glomerulonephritis, immune complex and antiglomerular basement membrane disease. Goodpasture's syndrome has pulmonary haemorrhage associated with glomerulonephritis and antiglomerular basement antibodies. Alternatively, idiopathic pulmonary haemosiderosis (IPH) is a disorder without immunological associations or renal disease. The aetiology of IPH is unknown and it eventually leads to lung fibrosis.

The typical findings are haemoptysis and anaemia with the chest radiograph showing diffuse alveolar consolidation.

Occupational lung diseases

Inhalational and other exposures to irritants in the workplace can cause lung disease. For example, some inhaled dusts can produce fibrosis in the lungs. Table 4.1 shows a list of common occupational lung diseases.

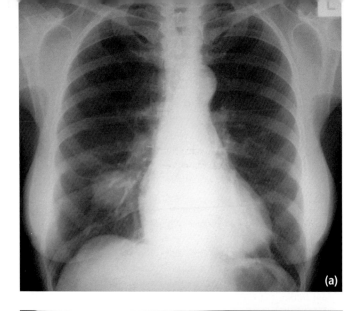

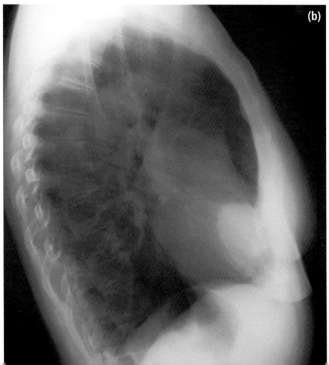

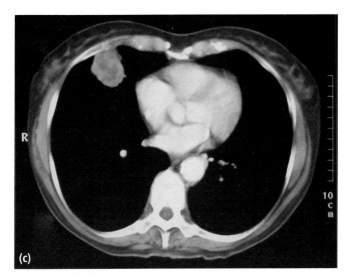

(c)

Fig. 4.5 Middle lobe tumour: (a) PA view; (b) lateral view; (c) CT scan

There is a 3.5 cm tumour in the anterior aspect of the medial segment of the middle lobe. It is clearly separated from the right heart border and not involved in any lung collapse. Vessels from the inferior part of the hilum are visible through the mass. (See Hilum overlay sign, Appendix 1.)

Justifiable questions to ask from the film are:

- Is the patient a smoker?
- Is there history or symptoms of any extrapulmonary primary tumour and are any previous films available for comparison?

Because there is a strong possibility that this is a malignant mass, signs of metastatic disease, such as hilar and mediastinal lymphadenopathy, pleural effusion or other lung nodules, need to be recognised. (See differential diagnosis of solitary pulmonary nodule, Appendix 2.) Note that the term 'coin lesion' is best avoided. Although it describes the shadow cast, it does not describe the three-dimensional structure.

Critical issues:

- If this is an isolated bronchogenic carcinoma (T2 N0 M0) and is surgically resected, the five-year survival is about 50%.
- If this is a solitary metastatic deposit, the common primary sources are likely to be colon, breast, renal, melanoma or testicular. The chance of a metastasis is very low if there is no history or symptoms of a primary tumour.
- The Fleischner Society recommends using the word 'nodule' for a lesion up to 3 cm in diameter and a 'mass' for a lesion greater than 3 cm in diameter. This distinction is not rigid for other authorities.

Table 4.1   Occupational lung diseases

Asbestos dust inhalation

- Pleural plaques
- Rounded atelectasis
- Pleural effusions
- Asbestosis
- Mesothelioma and carcinoma

Pneumoconiosis

- Silicosis → progressive massive fibrosis
- Coal workers' pneumoconiosis

Interstitial fibrosis (fibrosing alveolitis)

- Paraquat poisoning
- Asbestosis

Extrinsic allergic alveolitis

- Farmer's lung
- Bagassosis
- Humidifier fever

Bronchogenic carcinoma

- Asbestos
- Nickel, uranium, cadmium
- Passive smoking

Chemical pneumonitis

- Inhaled aerosols

Beryllium pneumopathy

- Acute: tracheobronchitis and pulmonary oedema
- Chronic: sarcoid-like

Asthma

There are over 150 chronic infiltrative lung diseases, with twelve diseases accounting for 90% of cases. These diseases are:

- usual interstitial pneumonia/idiopathic pulmonary fibrosis (UIP/IPF)
- asbestosis
- desquamative interstitial pneumonia/respiratory bronchiolitis–interstitial lung disease (DIP/RB–ILD)
- sarcoidosis
- silicosis
- extrinsic allergic alveolitis (EAA)
- pulmonary Langerhan's cell histiocytosis (PLCH)
- chronic eosinophilic pneumonia
- alveolar proteinosis
- lymphangitic metastases
- bronchiolitis obliterans with organising pneumonia (BOOP)
- non-specific interstitial pneumonia (NSIP).

Interstitial lung disease (see Fig. 4.6) can be differentiated based on CXR observations. These are listed in Table 4.2.

HRCT indications include normal CXR, pattern determination and localising the best biopsy site.

Table 4.2	Interstitial lung disease
CXR	**Disease**
Bibasal involvement	IPF, asbestosis, collagen vascular diseases
Mid and upper lung involvement	Sarcoidosis, silicosis, ankylosing spondylitis, PLCH
Pleural disease	Collagen vascular disease, asbestosis
Hilar lymphadenopathy	Sarcoidosis, malignancy
↓ Lung volumes	Most ILD
Preserved lung volumes	Lympangioleiomyomatosis, PLCH, sarcoidosis
Smokers	DIP, RB-ILD, PLCH

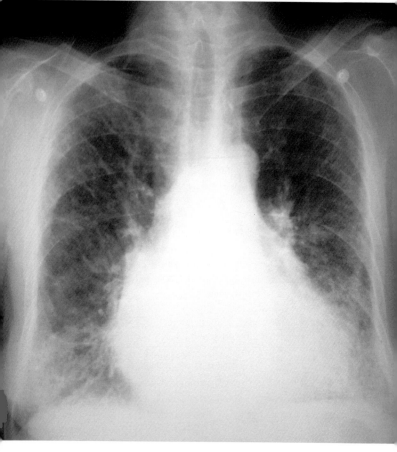

Fig. 4.6 Interstitial fibrosis: PA view

An increase in interstitial shadowing is seen involving all the zones with predominance in the lower zones. At this stage no major volume loss is evident.

It is important to check whether there are signs of previous asbestos exposure, such as pleural calcification. Also check whether there are signs of an erosive artropathy as rheumatoid arthritis could be a cause. With scleroderma, a dilated oesophagus may be visible.

Interstitial fibrosis is a cause of pulmonary hypertension and right heart failure.

Chapter 5
Cardiovascular disorders

The chest radiograph is the first and basic imaging investigation for cardiovascular disorders. There are a multitude of other imaging tests and imaging indications and protocols.

The heart size and shape need to be assessed first. Remember that a pericardial effusion can mimic cardiomegaly. Also, it is important to remember that the cardiothoracic ratio is only reliable on posteroanterior (PA) inspiratory films.

The heart shape is abnormal in congenital conditions such as dextrocardia (see Fig. 5.1), tetralogy of Fallot and Ebstein's anomaly but it is also important to assess the pulmonary vasculature for evidence of shunts.

Sometimes calcifications are visible in the cardiac shadow. They can occur in the valves, coronary arteries, left ventricular aneurysms (see Fig. 5.2) and in the pericardium. Pericardial calcification often, but not always, correlates with constrictive pericarditis.

Old valve prostheses can sometimes be visible but not the newer prostheses.

All introduced lines and catheters must be checked for their positions. Central lines should pass to the lower superior vena cava (SVC). Pulmonary artery catheters (Swan–Ganz catheters) should not be wedged into small branches. An atrial pacing wire should pass to the lateral wall of the right atrium, whereas the ventricular pacing wire should pass to the apex of the right ventricle. When line and catheter positions are being checked, ensure that there is no iatrogenic pneumothorax.

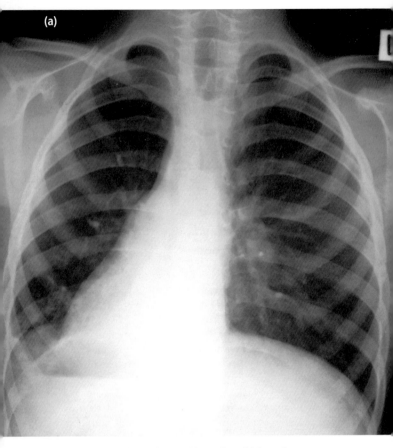

Fig. 5.1 Kartagener's syndrome: (a) PA view; (b) bronchogram
The frontal radiograph shows dextrocardia, an increase in markings at the right base due to bronchiectasis and collapse of the right lower lobe (a complication of the bronchiectasis and not part of the syndrome). Please note the gastric air bubble on the right indicating that the dextrocardia is not isolated but part of the situs inversus.

The dilated bronchi are demonstrated on the bronchogram.

Kartagener's syndrome is the triad of situs inversus (dextrocardia), bronchiectasis and paranasal sinusitis. About 50% of patients with ciliary dyskinesia have Kartagener's syndrome. About 20% of patients with dextrocardia have Kartagener's syndrome.

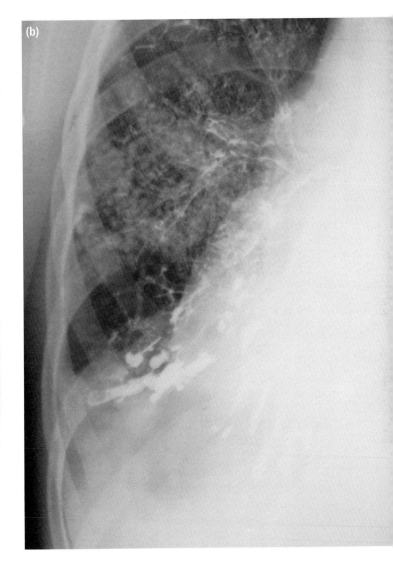

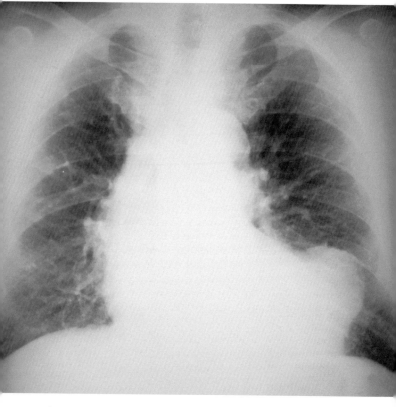

Fig. 5.2 Ventricular aneurysm: PA view

A very prominent bulge is seen on the left heart border due to a ventricular aneurysm. This type of aneurysm usually follows a myocardial infarct and is at risk of rupturing. Differential diagnostic possibilities include localised pericardial defect, cardiac tumour or adjacent pulmonary tumour (see Third mogul sign, Appendix 1).

Pulmonary oedema

Pulmonary oedema is the abnormal accumulation of extravascular water in the lung parenchyma.

Normally, there is a net outward filtration of fluid from the lung microvasculature to the perimicrovascular spaces. This small amount of fluid is removed by the pulmonary lymphatic vessels to keep the lungs dry. The lung dryness/wetness status is influenced by:

- capillary blood pressure
- plasma osmotic pressure
- capillary permeability
- alveolar surface tension (surfactant).

Pulmonary oedema is usually due to either elevated pulmonary venous pressure—'cardiogenic' oedema—or increased permeability of the alveolar-capillary membrane—'non-cardiogenic' oedema. *Hydrostatic pulmonary oedema* is probably a better term than 'cardiogenic' as the main causes are heart disease (increased capillary pressure), over-hydration (aggressive intravenous fluid therapy) or fluid retention (renal failure). In '*non-cardiogenic' pulmonary* oedema, there is some disruption of the capillary endothelium with leakage of fluid into the surrounding lung tissue. However, the oedema fluid is more proteinaceous than in hydrostatic oedema because the capillary injury permits the escape of large molecules as well as fluid.

Although traditionally pulmonary oedema has been classified as being either cardiogenic (hydrostatic) or non-cardiogenic (increased permeability), a better classification is into four types:

1. hydrostatic
2. permeability oedema without alveolar damage
3. permeability oedema with alveolar damage (ARDS)
4. mixed hydrostatic and permeability oedema.

Congestive left heart failure

There is a typical sequence of changes in the lungs as the left heart fails, from upper zone blood diversion to interstitial pulmonary oedema to alveolar pulmonary oedema.

The normal left atrial pressure or pulmonary venous pressure is less than 12 mmHg. As the heart fails, the pressures rise and produce the typical radiographic changes. The pressure rises in the pulmonary veins can be measured by wedging a pulmonary artery catheter (PAWP).

In the erect position, there is a hydrostatic difference in pressure between the apices and the bases; and in the supine position, between the anterior and posterior aspects. This difference in hydrostatic pressure needs to be added to the pulmonary venous pressure. It also explains why there is more flow to the lower zones and why the first changes occur here. Table 5.1 shows the features of left ventricular failure.

Table 5.1 **Features of left ventricular failure**
• Cardiomegaly (cardiac apex points downwards and outwards)
• Prominent central pulmonary arteries
• Signs of upper zone blood diversion and oedema
• Increase in width of the vascular pedicle

Upper zone blood diversion

In response to the elevated venous pressure (13–17 mmHg), arterial and venous constriction occurs in the lower zones, deviating blood flow to the upper zones (see Fig. 5.3). It is thought that the vasoconstriction is a reaction to early perivascular oedema.

This redistribution of blood flow causes the vessel diameters in the upper zones to be equal to or greater than the comparable lower zone vessels. Also, the upper zone vessels become wider than the accompanying bronchus (normally the upper zone artery should not exceed its bronchus in diameter). A confirmatory sign is that the vessels projected in the first anterior intercostal space exceed 3 mm in calibre.

Interstitial pulmonary oedema

With a further rise of the pulmonary venous pressure above 17 mmHg there is leakage of fluid into the interstitium thickening the alveolar walls and interlobular connective tissues. The radiologic signs of interstitial oedema are:

• Kerley lines (oedematous interlobular septa)
• perihilar haze (ground-glass appearance) due to oedema in the extensive interstitial space
• perivascular and peribronchial cuffing
• subpleural fluid accumulation giving the fissures a thickened appearance

- development of a pleural effusion, usually right sided, when the pressure is above 20 mmHg.

The pleural fluid represents transudation of fluid from the visceral pleural surface into the pleural space.

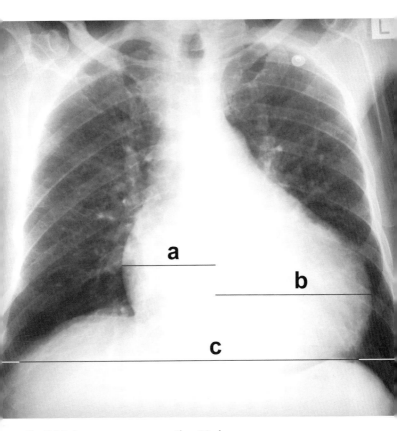

Fig. 5.3 Pulmonary venous congestion: PA view
The early sign of left heart failure is the shunting of blood into the upper zone vessels.
The cardiothoracic ratio is the total transverse diameter of the cardiac shadow and the internal diameter of the chest ($a + b : c$). In this case it is increased above 50%, also indicating that there is left heart failure.

Alveolar pulmonary oedema

When the pulmonary venous pressure rises above 20 mmHg, alveolar oedema fluid spills from the interstitium to the airspaces (see Figs 5.4, 5.5). Leakage occurs across the previously intact 'tight junctions' of the epithelial basement membrane. The signs of alveolar oedema are:

- confluent non-segmental shadows in a batwing/butterfly distribution
- air bronchogram sign (see Appendix 1)
- signs of interstitial oedema.

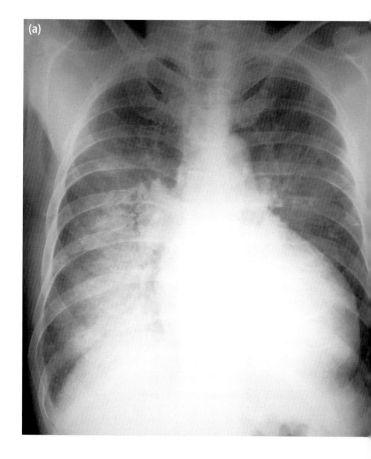
(a)

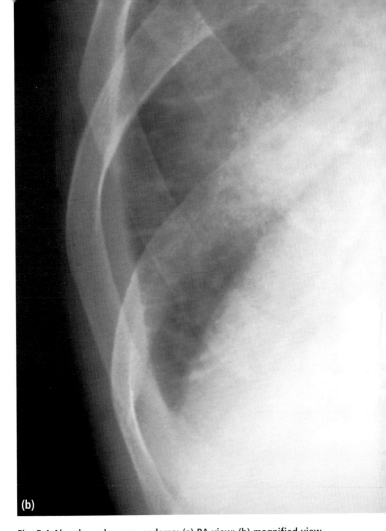

Fig. 5.4 Alveolar pulmonary oedema: (a) PA view; (b) magnified view
The transudate is filling the airspaces and causing the lung to be dense, mainly in a perihilar distribution.

Signs of interstitial pulmonary oedema are also present with transudate thickening the interlobular septa (Kerley B lines). A subpleural or lamellar effusion is also present. The lamellar effusion is a fluid collection in the loose connective tissue beneath the visceral pleura.

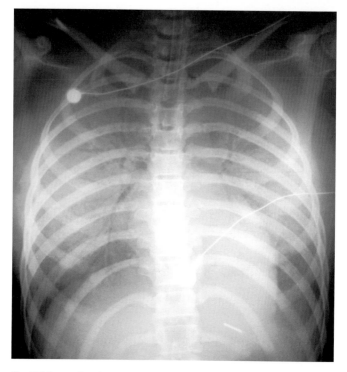

Fig. 5.5 Gross alveolar oedema: AP view
This radiograph shows diffuse and marked airspace filling caused by over-hydration intravenously. Note the normal-sized heart. Air bronchogram signs (see Appendix 1) are well demonstrated.

Airspace filling can be due to transudate (alveolar oedema), exudate (pneumonia), protein (alveolar proteinosis) or cells (alveolar cell carcinoma or lymphoma).

Compartments

The interstitial compartment becomes oedematous first in cardiogenic oedema and therefore may be present without alveolar oedema. However, if alveolar oedema is present, then the interstitial compartment must also be oedematous. Therefore, the signs of alveolar oedema overlay the signs of interstitial oedema.

In increased-permeability oedema, the fluid spills directly into the alveolar spaces and therefore the interstitium may not be oedematous.

Speed

With treatment, pulmonary oedema can clear rapidly from the lungs. Even so, there can be a 'lag phase' between improving capillary wedge pressure and radiographic resolution. The exception is 'uraemic' pulmonary oedema, which is fibrinous and in which clearing may be very delayed.

Distribution

The distribution of alveolar oedema depends on:
• the patient's posture (e.g. unilateral oedema if the patient is lying on his/her side)
• other lung pathology (e.g. emphysema).

In chronic lung disease there is regional destruction of vasculature with redistribution of blood flow to uninvolved areas which are potential sites for the oedema. Therefore, an 'atypical' distribution is seen.

Central distribution of alveolar oedema occurs because there is more interstitium, a less adequate lymphatic system and less respiratory compression.

Chronicity

In chronic heart or lung disease, the radiologic changes may occur at higher pressures because of hypertrophy of the lymphatic vessels and adaptations in the microvasculature.

Distinguishing features

Sometimes there are clues to differentiate between cardiogenic and other types of oedema. In cardiogenic oedema, the heart is enlarged and septal lines are common, whereas in increased-permeability oedema the heart size is normal and septal lines are uncommon. In hydrostatic oedema, due to massive intravenous fluid overload, the heart size will not be increased.

Lung volumes

Lung volumes are decreased in pulmonary oedema because of reduced lung compliance.

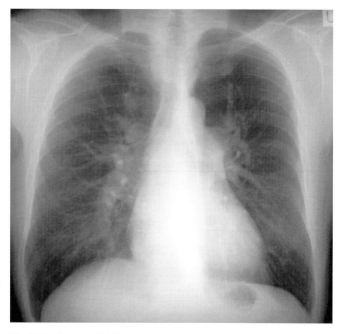

Fig. 5.6 Atrial septal defect (ASD): PA view

In this case of ASD, there is an uncomplicated left-to-right shunt without cardiac enlargement. Enlargement of all the pulmonary vessels, both central and peripheral, in all zones is present, secondary to the increased pulmonary blood flow.

The right heart border (right lateral margin of the right atrium) is prominent. The cardiac apex is becoming elevated, suggesting right ventricular enlargement. The distended pulmonary trunk is causing a bulge below the aortic knuckle. The aortic knuckle is small relative to the pulmonary artery trunk, reflecting the decreased left ventricular output.

Pulmonary arterial over-circulation does not become apparent on chest radiographs until there is a ratio of shunt flow : systemic flow of 2 : 1. The over-circulation causes pulmonary hypertension when the pressures are greater than 30/15 mmHg (normal pulmonary arterial pressure is 25/10 mmHg). Only with longstanding severe shunts where the pulmonary artery pressure increases above the systemic pressure does reversal of the shunt occur (Eisenmenger's syndrome). In Eisenmenger's syndrome there is very marked dilatation of the central pulmonary arteries and abrupt pruning of the peripheral arteries as a sign of the increased vascular resistance.

Note that the prominent arteries in this case have sharp margins. This is an important distinguishing feature between a shunt and pulmonary venous hypertension.

Further reading

Web pages

There are several teaching files and other resources online:

<http://www.chestX-ray.com>

<http://www.eurorad.org>—go to Chest Imaging

<http://www.sbu.ac.uk/~dirt/museum/g-topics.html>

<http://www.vh.org>

<http://www.mypacs.net>

<http://www.med.wayne.edu/diagRadiology/TeachingFile.html>

<http://www.uhrad.com>—go to the section on Body Imaging

<http://www.ibiblio.org/jksmith/UNC-Radiology-Webserver/
mainmenu.html>—go to Teaching File

<http://www.auntminnie.com>—go to Reference and then Thoracic
Radiology

<http://www.brighamrad.harvard.edu/fire>

<http://www.mds.qmw.ac.uk/radiology/>

<http://www.ctisus.org>

<http://www.meddean.luc.edu/lumen/MedEd/medicine/pulmonar/
cxr/cxr.htm>

Bibliography

Armstrong P, Wilson AG, Dee P, Hansell D. Imaging of diseases of the chest. 3rd edn. London: Mosby, 2000.

Briggs GM. Chest imaging: indications and interpretation. *Med J Aust* 1997;166:555–60.

Collins J, Stern E. Chest radiology: The essentials. Baltimore: Lippincott, Williams & Wilkins, 1999.

Felson B. Chest radiography. Philadelphia: WB Saunders Co., 1973.

Figley MM, Gerdes AJ, Ricketts HJ. Radiographic aspects of pulmonary embolism. *Semin Roentgenol* 1967;2:389–405.

Fraser R, Pare JAP, Pare PD et al. Diagnosis of diseases of the chest. 3rd edn. Philadelphia: WB Saunders Co., 1998.

Freundlich IM, Bragg DG. A radiologic approach to diseases of the chest. 2nd edn. Baltimore: Williams & Wilkins, 1997.

Gurney JW, Winer-Muram HT. Pocket radiologist chest top 100 diagnoses. Salt Lake City: WB Saunders Co., 2002.

McLoud TC. Thoracic radiology: The requisites. St Louis: Mosby, 1998.

Mergo PJ. Imaging of the chest. Baltimore: Lippincott, Williams & Wilkins, 2002.

Sutton D, ed. A textbook of radiology and imaging. 3rd edn. Edinburgh: Churchill Livingstone, 1980.

Glossary references

Tuddenham WJ. Glossary of terms for thoracic radiology: recommendations of the Nomenclature Committee of the Fleischner Society. *AJR* 1984;143:509–17.

Austin JHM, Muller NL, Friedman PJ et al. Glossary of terms for CT of the lungs: recommendations of the Nomenclature Committee of the Fleischner Society. *Radiology* 1996;200:327–31.

Webb RW, Muller NL, Naidich DP. Illustrated glossary in high-resolution computed tomography terms. In: High resolution CT of the lung. 3rd edn. Baltimore: Lippincott, Williams & Wilkins, 2001: 599–618.

Signs in thoracic radiology

A 'sign' in radiology refers to an abnormal radiological finding that suggests a specific disease process or possible group of disorders. A 'pattern' refers to a collection of radiological findings. The basic signs in chest radiology are:

- air bronchogram
- atelectasis
- bronchial wall thickening
- calcification
- cavitation
- consolidation
- ground-glass opacity
- mass/nodule
- reticular shadowing.

The following signs are used in thoracic radiology. Because of overlap and to help with understanding of disease processes, CT signs have been included for completeness.

acinar pattern A collection of poorly defined or partly confluent opacities. They are 4–8 mm in diameter and together produce an inhomogeneous shadow. Similar terms are rosette pattern and acinose pattern (used specifically for endobronchial spread of tuberculosis).

air bronchogram sign The bronchus is visible as an air-filled structure surrounded by consolidated or collapsed lung. The most common causes are pneumonia and alveolar pulmonary oedema. When associated with collapse, its presence implies that the bronchus is not obstructed at its origin. Pulmonary lymphoma and alveolar cell carcinoma are tumours that can have a characteristic air bronchogram sign. See B6 bronchus sign.

air crescent (meniscus) sign A radiolucent crescent becomes apparent at the periphery of a pulmonary mass lesion or when an area of pneumonia undergoes necrosis and cavitates. It most commonly occurs with an intracavitary fungus ball but can also be seen in hydatid cyst, lung abscess, haematoma and tumours.

anterior sulcus sign Also known as the 'double diaphragm sign'. It shows as a lucency over the upper quadrant when a pneumo-thorax is present in a supine patient. The free air lies in the anterior diaphragmatic sulcus, which is the uppermost portion of the thorax when the patient is supine. When detected, further views are required to establish the presence of the pneumothorax.

aortic nipple sign The left intercostal vein may drain anteriorly across the aortic arch to the innominate vein. This vein projects as a nipple on the aortic knuckle.

atelectasis Collapse and volume loss are synonymous terms.

B6 bronchus sign The B6 bronchus supplies the apical segment of the right lower lobe. When this segment is involved with consolidation or non-obstructing atelectasis, the B6 bronchus which passes anteroposteriorly is visible, projected just above the right hilum on the frontal view.

batwing distribution Colloquially called bat's wing shadowing. See Butterfly shadow.

beaded septum sign Small nodules may appear as a row of beads at a septum or fissure as an indication of lymphatic involvement. Lymphangitic carcinomatosis and sarcoidosis are the two main causes of this appearance.

big rib sign The ribs on the side of the patient closest to the X-ray tube (i.e. furthest from the film cassette) are magnified on the lateral CXR. This helps localisation of disease or a hemidiaphragm to the right or left side.

black bronchus sign The air within the bronchus is obviously blacker compared to the ground-glass opacity in the lungs. In normal lungs the blackness is only marginal.

black pleura sign The pleura appears as a lucent line between the calcified pulmonary infiltrate (microlithiasis) and the adjacent ribs.

bronchial wall thickening Oedema, inflammatory cells or neoplastic cells infiltrate the peribronchial interstitial space. (See differential diagnosis of peribronchial cuffing, Appendix 2.)

bulging fissure sign If a consolidated lobe is swollen and enlarged, the fissure becomes displaced. The classic pneumonic process causing this is *Klebsiella* pneumonia (Friedlander's bacillus); but it can also occur with *Haemophilus influenzae*, pneumococcal and tuberculous pneumonias.

butterfly (batwing) shadow This is the classic perihilar distribution of acute alveolar pulmonary oedema with a bilateral symmetric pattern. The central portion of the lungs shows shadowing (airspace filling) with the outer lung aerated. The reason/cause/mechanism may be due to the better lymphatic drainage in the outer portions of the lungs or the better aeration peripherally during the respiratory cycle.

calcification Deposition of calcium salts within a structure rendering it visible on X-ray examination.

cavitation A cavity forms in an area of consolidation when necrosis occurs. Air enters the cavity when there is communication with the bronchial tree.

cervicothoracic sign This sign helps to indicate whether an upper mediastinal mass lies anteriorly or posteriorly. If a mass lies anteriorly, its upper border disappears as it approaches the clavicles. Because the posterior lung passes more highly, any posterior mediastinal mass outlined by the adjacent lung will show up above the clavicles.

cœur en sabot sign The French '*cœur en sabot*' literally means the curved toe portion of a wooden shoe. It is the shape of the heart in tetralogy of Fallot where the apex points upwards and outwards due to the right ventricular hypertrophy.

comet tail sign On CT images, bronchovascular structures are twisted into a juxtapleural mass of 'rounded atelectasis' with the tail pointing towards the hilum.

consolidation Filling of the airspaces with abnormal material such as transudate, exudate, cells or protein. Consolidated lung characteristically appears dense and shows the bronchi as air-filled tubular structures (see Air bronchogram sign) but obscures the underlying vessels.

continuous diaphragm sign The central junction between the two hemidiaphragms is normally not seen because of the heart. In cases of pneumomediastinum where gas is present extrapleurally between the heart and diaphragm, the central portion is also visualised.

corona radiata sign Numerous radiating strands around the edge of a nodule which has a sunburst appearance. It usually indicates a bronchial carcinoma but rarely can be seen with infectious granulomas.

costal cartilage sign In men, the upper and lower portions of the costal cartilage become calcified first adjacent to the bony rib ends. In women, the central part of the costal cartilage adjacent to the rib calcifies first.

crow's feet sign Bands of fibrosis radiate from a visceral pleural focus into the lung.

CT angiogram sign Pulmonary vessels are visualised on contrast-enhanced CT scanning against a background of relatively low attenuation material. It is seen with pneumonia, alveolar pulmonary oedema, alveolar cell carcinoma and lymphoma.

D sign A loculated pleural effusion will give a homogeneous peripheral opacity in the shape of a 'D'. When projected over the thoracic spine on the lateral CXR, it has been called the 'forward S' sign.

deep sulcus sign Pleural air collections in the supine patient lie anteriorly because this is the uppermost portion of the supine chest. The collected air makes the lateral costophrenic angle look deeper and the hemidiaphragm appears less dense. The signs of an apical pneumothorax are not present.

double contour sign The right heart border (right lateral margin of the right atrium) is normally outlined by the medial segment of the middle lobe. When the left atrium is enlarged, it bulges posteriorly and then at its side. The double contour is either the right margin of the left atrium lying densely behind the right heart border or, when massively dilated, extending beyond the right atrium.

double diaphragm sign When there is a pneumothorax in a supine patient, the anterior sulcus and the dome of the true hemi-diaphragm may be visualised simultaneously. See anterior sulcus sign and deep sulcus sign.

eggshell calcification Hilar lymph nodes which have peripheral ring of calcification. Classically occurs with silicosis (5%) but can be mimicked by sarcoidosis, healed tuberculosis and treated lymphoma.

fallen lung sign This rare sign can occur if there is a bronchial fracture but the vascular pedicle remains intact. There is a pneumothorax and the lung sags downwards on an erect film and not inwards towards the hilum.

feeding vessel sign A distinct vessel leading to the apex of a peripheral area of consolidation.

flat waist sign The contours of the aortic knuckle and pulmonary artery become flattened in complete collapse of the left lower lobe due to leftward displacement and rotation of the heart.

Fleischner sign The hilum appears plump when there is a bulky embolus obstructing the main pulmonary artery at the hilum. This is highlighted by the decreased pulmonary artery branches beyond it.

floating hilum sign The 'clear space' between hilar lymph-adenopathy and the mediastinum distinguishes it from mediastinal lymphadenopathy.

gloved finger shadow sign When bronchi become ectatic and filled with mucus, their tubular appearances resemble gloved fingers. One type is the 'toothpaste shadow' in allergic broncho-pulmonary aspergillosis, where a band opacity of mucoid impaction points to the hilum.

Golden S sign See S sign of Golden.

ground-glass opacity This term describes a hazy increase in lung density. It must be subtle and not dense enough to obscure visualisation of the pulmonary vessels. It can be caused by airspace disease, interstitial thickening and even deflation.

halo sign A dense focal area of consolidation is surrounded by a halo of ground-glass opacity on CT scanning. It can be seen with haemorrhagic nodules such as Kaposi's sarcoma and Wegener's granulomatosis; and also seen in early invasive pulmonary aspergillosis.

Hampton's hump sign A pulmonary infarct appears as a homogeneous wedge-shaped opacity with its base against the visceral pleura and a rounded apex directed towards the hilum. See Melting ice cube sign.

hanging drop heart The heart may appear normal in size, even though it is compromised, in chronic obstructive pulmonary disease by the hyperinflation of the lungs and depression of the hemidiaphragms.

head-cheese sign A mixture of lung attenuation with geographic areas of normal lung, ground-glass opacity and mosaic perfusion are seen on high-resolution CT. It resembles a sausage made from the head of a hog. It usually indicates infiltrative and obstructive disease. The common causes are sarcoidosis, hypersensitivity pneumonitis and infective bronchiolitis.

hilum overlay sign If a structure is projected over the hilum, yet is separated from it, the hilar shape remains visible because of the adjacent aerated lung. This is different when a mass involves the hilum and the normal hilar configuration and outline are lost.

Hoffman–Rigler sign This is a superseded and complicated sign which indicates left ventricular enlargement on the lateral view by comparing the posterior border of the left ventricle to the inferior vena cava position.

honeycomb shadowing Cystic airspaces are apparent as ring shadows between coarse reticular shadowing. It implies destruction and fibrosis of alveolar walls and causes traction bronchiectasis.

hyperlucent hemithorax sign This sign can be due to a number of factors and occurs when there is unilateral hyperlucency or increased 'blackness'. It could be due to rotation, mastectomy, pneumothorax, previous surgery or reduced pulmonary vessels.

iceberg sign The top of thoraco-abdominal masses may be visible where they are in contact with the aerated lower lobes; but the lack of a lower border suggests that most of the mass lies in the abdomen. This sign can be seen in thoraco-abdominal aneurysms, oesophagogastric tumours, azygos continuations of the inferior vena cava and also retroperitoneal tumours extending into the thorax.

interface sign Nodular irregularity of bronchoarterial bundles in association with the beaded septum sign. Occurs in lymphangitis, carcinomatosis and sarcoidosis.

juxtaphrenic peak sign In right upper lobe collapse, a small triangular shadow may obscure the dome of the right hemi-diaphragm.

Kerley lines First described in 1933 by radiologist Dr Peter Kerley, who thought that they were due to engorged lymphatics. In 1951 he categorised the three patterns into A, B and C lines. These are septal lines that are thickened by fluid accumulation, cellular infiltration or connective tissue proliferation within the interlobular septa. They can be acute and transient, or chronic, due to lymphatic obstruction or fibrosis.

- Kerley A lines are straight 2–6 cm lines, 1 mm in thickness, located in a radiating fashion midway between the hilum and pleura. They appear to cross over the bronchoarterial bundles.
- Kerley B lines are 1 cm long, perpendicular to the lateral pleural surface. They are usually seen just above the costophrenic angles.
- Kerley C lines are a fine network of superimposed Kerley B lines seen 'en face'.
- Kreel's D lines are seen on the lateral CXR.

luftsichel sign Occurs with left upper lobe collapse and is the paramediastinal translucency projected above the left hilum. It is derived from the German words '*Luft*' (air) and '*Sichel*' (sickle). The lucency is the aerated apex of the lower lobe positioned between the mediastinum and the collapsed left upper lobe. Originally it was thought to be due to herniation of the right lung across the mid-line. It needs to be distinguished from a loculated medial pneumothorax.

mass A discrete opacity greater than 3 cm in size.

melting ice cube sign A resolving pulmonary infarct maintains its homogeneity and wedge shape, unlike pneumonia, which resolves in a patchy manner.

meniscus sign A curved upper margin of a peripheral homogeneous opacity suggests a pleural effusion. It is due to the tapering split between the visceral and parietal pleural layers.

miliary pattern A collection of tiny discrete pulmonary opacities that are generally uniform in size (2 mm or less) and widespread in distribution.

mosaic pattern Regional differences in lung density are seen when there are areas of ground-glass opacity and areas of hypodense lung. The three basic causes are infiltrative lung disease, small airways disease and occlusive vascular disease. Constrictive obliterative bronchiolitis and multiple pulmonary emboli will produce hypodense lung with the blood shunted into the 'normal' ground-glass lung. These two processes can be distinguished by expiratory scans. Similar terms are mosaic perfusion and mosaic oligaemia.

mucoid impaction The presence of thick tenacious mucus within an airway produces band Y- or V-shaped opacities.

nodule A nodule is a mass less than 3 cm in size but the term can also be used interchangeably with mass. A nodular pattern is produced when rounded lesions accumulate in the interstitium.

Nordenstrom's sign Lingular atelectasis which is associated with left lower lobe collapse.

oesophageal tube displacement sign The oesophagus and oesophageal tube are displaced by haematoma when there is an aortic tear following trauma. Emergency aortography is indicated.

paratracheal stripe sign On a PA CXR, the right paratracheal stripe should be thin and becomes thickened with adjacent lymphadenopathy or haemorrhage. On the lateral CXR, the posterior margin of the trachea should be thin and, if it is thickened, adjacent pathology should be suspected.

pleural tail sign A line shadow connecting a peripheral nodule to the pleura. Also known as a pleuropulmonary tail. This sign is not specific and is seen with a variety of lesions, both malignant and benign, particularly granulomas.

reticular shadowing Fine, medium or coarse irregular linear opacities due to interstitial thickening. When combined with nodular opacities it is described as a reticulonodular pattern.

ring around the artery sign A well-defined lucent ring is seen around the right pulmonary artery on the lateral film in the presence of a pneumomediastinum.

S sign of Golden A right paramediastinal opacity with a margin of a reversed S is seen with a hilar malignant tumour obstructing the right upper lobe bronchus, causing collapse. The affected fissure has a central convexity because of the mass itself and a distal concave shape as a result of the collapse.

saber sheath trachea sign The intrathoracic trachea shape can change in chronic obstructive pulmonary disease and can have a narrowed coronal width. Also called a scabbard trachea.

sail sign The shadow of the normal thymus is seen projecting laterally beyond the rest of the mediastinum. It is seen in neonates and young children and must not be confused with a consolidated right upper lobe.

scimitar sign A curved band resembling a Turkish scimitar is the shadow produced by an anomalous pulmonary vein coursing through the lung and draining into a subdiaphragmatic inferior vena cava.

sentinel lines sign These lines can occur at the lung bases and be a sign of adjacent lower lobe volume loss. It is thought that they are due to bronchial kinking with distal atelectasis. They must be distinguished from other causes of plate-like atelectasis and septal lines. See Nordenstrom's sign.

shaggy heart sign The pulmonary and pleural changes in asbestosis may partially blur the cardiac outline.

shifting granuloma sign If the position of a nodule shifts between examinations, it implies loss of volume in one part of the lung: an internal marker of atelectasis.

shrinking lungs Diaphragm dysfunction can occur in systemic lupus erythematous. The lungs lose volume as the diaphragm rises.

signet ring sign This is a sign of bronchiectasis and is seen when the segmental bronchus is larger in diameter than the accompanying pulmonary artery.

silhouette sign More accurately this should be called the 'loss of silhouette sign'. Whenever there is loss of a mediastinal border or diaphragmatic outline, it indicates that aerated lung is no longer outlining it. For instance, if there is loss of outline of the aortic knob it implies that there is a lesion or consolidation in the apicoposterior segment of the left upper lobe adjacent to the aortic knob.

snowman sign An unusual cardiac configuration due to total anomalous pulmonary venous drainage. The bottom of the snowman is the enlargement of the right atrium and ventricle. The top of the snowman is the superior mediastinal enlargement caused by the total anomalous pulmonary vein drainage into the superior vena cava or azygos vein. Other terms used to describe the cardiac shape are 'cottage loaf' or 'figure of 8'.

spinnaker sign Loculated air in a pneumomediastinum pushes the thymus into the shape of a spinnaker.

split pleura sign Normally the opposed parietal and visceral pleural are not separated. Loculated fluid can, however, separate or split the thickened pleural envelope. The loculated fluid is usually lenticular in shape and infected. The subpleural fat adjacent to the parietal fluid can be thickened and oedematous. This sign can be useful in differentiating an empyema from a lung abscess. It can also be seen with haemothorax and talc pleurodesis.

third mogul sign The third mogul is any abnormal protuberance on the left heart border. It could be due to an adjacent lesion or a large left atrial appendage. The first mogul is the aortic knob; the second mogul is the left main pulmonary artery; the fourth mogul is the cardiac apex.

thymic wave sign Impressions from the costochondral junctions may be seen on the normal thymic outline on the frontal film. This sign is not seen in thymic tumours or other anterior mediastinal masses.

tramline sign Parallel lines from ectatic bronchi which may also be thickened from chronic infections.

tree-in-bud sign Peripheral small centrilobular nodules are connected to linear branching opacities (terminal bronchioles) that resemble a tree in bud. This pattern is seen on thin-section CT but is not visible on chest radiographs. With endobronchial spread of disease, the terminal bronchiole become dilated and impacted with mucus and pus. It is most commonly seen in atypical *Mycobacterium* infection (NTM).

upper triangle sign A triangular shadow is seen on the frontal radiograph resembling right upper lobe collapse when, in fact, there is collapse of the right lower lobe. It is caused by the rightward displacement of the upper mediastinum.

vanishing heart sign The margins of the heart become obscured in massive alveolar microlithiasis.

vertebral fade-off sign There is decreasing density posteriorly on the lateral radiograph from the upper thoracic spine to the very lowest thoracic spine at the diaphragm. The vertebral fade-off sign occurs with increased density due to overlying lung disease (e.g. lower lobe collapse).

waterfall sign Upper lobe fibrosis will elevate the hila. This causes the infrahilar pulmonary vessels to course downward more vertically than normal.

waterlily sign Hydatid cyst membranes floating on an air–fluid level indicate that the cyst has ruptured into a bronchus.

Westermark's sign There is relative lucency of a portion of lung distal to a large vessel embolus due to local oligaemia. This may be associated with enlargement of the ipsilateral main pulmonary artery (Fleischner sign). This sign can also occur with neoplastic destruction of a central pulmonary artery.

Appendix 2
Lists of causes and differential diagnoses

Causes of symptoms

Chest pain	Myocardial infarction
	Aortic dissection
	Pneumothorax
	Rib fractures
	Pneumonia
	Oesophageal rupture
	Pulmonary embolus

Dyspnoea	Pulmonary embolus
	Emphysema
	Interstitial fibrosis
	Pneumothorax, pleural effusion
	Tracheal compression
	Anaemia
	Pulmonary oedema
	Asthma
	Diaphragm palsy
	Airway foreign body

Haemoptysis	Pulmonary embolus
	Goodpasture's syndrome
	Bronchiectasis
	Lung carcinoma
	Tuberculosis
	Coagulopathy

Cough	Pneumonia
	Lung carcinoma
	Tracheal compression
	Chronic bronchitis
	Bronchiectasis
	Gastro-oesophageal reflux
	Goitre

Wheezing	Asthma
	Foreign body
	Pulmonary oedema
	Pulmonary eosinophilia

Normal CXR and dyspnoea	Pulmonary embolism
	Pneumocystis carinii pneumonia

Women in labour with dyspnoea and shock	Acute cardiogenic oedema
	Amniotic fluid embolism
	Massive gastric aspiration

Mediastinum

Anterior mediastinal masses (5Ts)	Thyroid
	Thymus
	Teratoma
	Terrible lymphoma
	Tortuous vessel
Middle mediastinal masses	Aortic arch aneurysm
	Bronchogenic cyst
	Hiatal hernia
	Lymphadenopathy
Posterior mediastinal masses	Neurogenic tumour
	Aneurysm of descending aorta
	Paraspinal lesion
	Extramedullary haemopoeisis
	Haematoma
	Lateral meningocoele
Shift of mediastinum to side of pathology	Collapsed lung segments/lobe
	Surgical removal of lung segments/lobe
	Hypoplasia of lung segments/lobe
Mediastinal shift to side opposite pathology	Large pleural mass or effusion
	Tension pneumothorax
	Foreign body (endobronchial—'ball valve')
	Bullae
	Diaphragmatic rupture/herniation
Pneumomediastinum in childhood	Airway foreign body
	Asthma
	Pharyngeal perforation
	Oesophageal perforation
	Membranous croup

Cardiac

Pulmonary arterial hypertension	
Precapillary	Chronic thromboemboli
	Chronic lung disease:
	• Emphysema
	• Chronic bronchitis
	• Interstitial fibrosis
	• Pleural fibrothorax
	Pulmonary vasculitis
	Eisenmenger's syndrome
	Primary pulmonary hypertension
Over-circulation	Atrial septal defect (ASD)
	Patent ductus arteriosus (PDA)
	Ventricular septal defect (VSD)
Postcapillary	Left ventricular failure
	Mitral valve disease
Hypoventilation	Obesity
	Sleep apnoea
	High altitude
	Chest wall deformity
Enlarged central pulmonary arteries	Pulmonary hypertension
	Post-stenotic dilatation
	Aneurysm
Redistribution of blood flow	Pulmonary venous hypertension
	Chronic obstructive pulmonary disease
	Pulmonary emboli
Left-to-right shunts	ASD
	VSD
	PDA

Cardiac (cont.)

Right-to-left shunts	Fallot's tetralogy Transposition of great vessels Eisenmenger's syndrome
Prominent ascending aorta ± arch	Aneurysm Aortic valve disease Atherosclerosis Coarctation Homocystinuria Marfan's syndrome PDA Pseudocoarctation Syphilitic aortitis Takayasu's arteritis Tetralogy of Fallot
Gross cardiac enlargement	Pericardial effusion Cardiomyopathy Valvular heart disease Ebstein's anomaly
Small heart	Emphysema (hanging drop heart) Addison's disease Dehydration Constrictive pericarditis Malnutrition Senile atrophy

Diaphragm

Elevated hemi-diaphragm	Normal variant (eventration, thinning) Splinting of diaphragm (acute abdominal or thoracic conditions) Elevation, secondary to lobar collapse Subpulmonary effusion Phrenic nerve paralysis Raised intra-abdominal pressure Diaphragmatic rupture/herniation Hemiplegia Gaseous distension of stomach (left)
Small lungs	Expiration Interstitial fibrosis Bilateral lobar collapse Bilateral elevated diaphragms Obesity Ascites Term pregnancy

Hila

Hilar lymph-adenopathy	Sarcoid
	Metastases
	Lymphoma
	Primary tuberculosis (TB)
	Infectious mononucleosis
	DD large pulmonary arteries
Unilateral hilar enlargement	Central bronchogenic carcinoma
	Metastatic lymphadenopathy
	Lymphoma
	Inflammatory lymphadenopathy
	Pulmonary embolism (Fleischner sign)
	Blocked contralateral pulmonary artery
Hilar eggshell calcification	Silicosis
	Sarcoidosis
	Lymphoma following radiotherapy
	Embolism

Pleura

Pleural calcification	Previous pleural TB
	Previous empyema
	Previous haemothorax
	Asbestos plaques
Pleural effusion	Transudate (protein < 3 g/dL):
	• Cardiac failure
	• Hypoalbuminaemia
	• Renal failure
	• Meig's syndrome
	• Peritoneal dialysis
	Exudate (protein > 3 g/dL):
	• Infection
	• Malignancy
	• Pulmonary embolus
	• Collagen diseases
	• Subphrenic abscess
	• Pancreatitis
	• Asbestos
	Haemorrhagic:
	• Trauma
	• Thoracotomy
	• Pulmonary infarct
	Chylous:
	• Obstructed thoracic duct
	• Lymphangio-leiomyomatosis (LAM)
Acute abdominal disease with pleural effusions	Pancreatitis
	Subphrenic abscess
	Perinephric abscess
	Trauma
	Leaking aneurysm
	Incarcerated diaphragmatic hernia
	Amoebic abscess

Pleura (cont.)

Pneumothorax	Spontaneous:
	• Apical blebs
	• Chronic obstructive pulmonary disease
	• Asthma
	• Cavitating pneumonia
	• Cystic fibrosis
	• Interstitial fibrosis
	• Pleural metastases
	• Pulmonary Langerhans cell histiocytosis (PLCH)
	• LAM/tuberous sclerosus
	• Catamenial pneumothorax
	• Connective tissue disorders
	• Pneumo-mediastinum extension
	• Pneumo-peritoneum extension
	• Bronchopleural fistula
	Traumatic:
	• Blunt or penetrating injury
	• Thoracotomy
	• Pleural aspiration
	• Percutaneous lung biopsy
	• Transbronchial lung biopsy
	• Central venous line insertion
	• Barotrauma

Lungs

Multiple pulmonary calcifications	Infection:
	• TB
	• Histoplasmosis, coccidioidomycosis
	• Chicken pox
	Metastases
	Mitral valve disease
	Alveolar microlithiasis
	Hyperparathyroidism
Ground glass on CXR	Acute symptoms:
	• Oedema
	• Haemorrhage
	• Infection
	• Acute interstitial pneumonia
	Chronic symptoms:
	• Hypersensitivity pneumonia
	• Usual interstitial pneumonia
	• Non-specific interstitial pneumonia
	• Desquamative interstitial pneumonia/respiratory bronchiolitis (RB-ILD)
	• Alveolar proteinosis (PAP)
Increased density of a hemithorax	Consolidation
	Pleural effusion
	Collapse
	Carcinoma, mesothelioma
	Post-pneumonectomy
	Fibrothorax
	Haemorrhage

Lungs (cont.)

Types of pulmonary collapse	Obstructive Passive atelectasis Adhesive atelectasis Cicatrising atelectasis
Collapse (lung, lobar, segmental)	Mucus plug (postoperative, asthma) Bronchogenic neoplasm Foreign body Endotracheal tube down bronchus Extrinsic lymph node compression Stricture: • post-inflammatory • post-radiotherapy
Alveolar filling (consolidation)	Acute—infection, haemorrhage, oedema Chronic—alveolar cell carcinoma, alveolar proteinosis
Lobar pneumonia	*Streptococcus pneumoniae* (commonest) *Klebsiella pneumoniae* (bulging fissures) *Staphylococcus aureus* TB
Antibiotic-resistant cavitary pneumonia	TB Atypical mycobacteria Nocardia Fungal pneumonia Sequestrated lung

Lungs (cont.)

Non-thrombotic pulmonary emboli	Septic emboli Catheter embolism Fat embolism syndrome Venous air embolism Amniotic fluid embolism Tumour embolism Talc embolism Vertebroplasty cement Rare: iodinated oil, mercury, cotton, hydatid
Septic pulmonary emboli	Tricuspid valve endocarditis Infected catheters and pacemaker wires Peripheral septic thrombophlebitis Intravenous drug abuse Organ transplants
Fat embolism syndrome	Trauma Haemoglobinopathy (sickle cell disease) Severe burns Soft tissue injuries Diabetes mellitus Pancreatitis Severe infection Neoplasms Osteomyelitis Blood transfusion Cardiopulmonary bypass Altitude decompression Suction lipectomy Renal transplantation Alcoholism Inhalational anaesthesia

Lungs (cont.)

Lucent lung fields	Technique
	Chronic obstructive airways disease
	Asthma
	Upper respiratory tract obstruction
	Acute bronchiolitis
	Pulmonary oligogaemia— right to left shunt, pulmonary artery stenosis, pulmonary emboli, primary pulmonary arterial hypertension
Unilateral hypertrans-lucency	Chest wall:
	• Mastectomy
	• Scoliosis
	• Polio
	• Poland's syndrome (unilateral absent pectoral muscle)
	Pulmonary:
	• Unilateral bullae
	• Compensatory hyperinflation
	• Swyer–James/ MacLeod's syndrome
	• Unilateral major embolus
	• Congenital lobar emphysema
	• Obstructive hyperaeration
	Pleura:
	• Pneumothorax
	• Contralateral pleural effusion (supine film)
	Rotation

Lungs (cont.)

Cystic lung disease	Emphysema
	Cystic bronchiectasis
	LAM/tuberous sclerosis
	Cystic metastases
	Wegener's granulomatosis
	Pneumocystis carinii pneumonia
	Septic pulmonary emboli
	Interstitial fibrosis (honeycombing)
	Papillomatosis
Increased interstitial markings	Interstitial pulmonary oedema
	Chronic bronchitis
	Lymphangitis carcinomatosa
	Pneumocystis carinii pneumonia
	Interstitial fibrosis (drugs, connective tissue disease, asbestosis, idiopathic)
	Sarcoidosis
Interstitial fibrosis	Idiopathic (most common cause)
	Collagen disease (rheumatoid, scleroderma, systemic lupus erythematosus [SLE])
	Asbestosis, silicosis
	Drugs (amiodarone, nitrofurantoin, cytotoxics, methysergide)
	Paraquat poisoning

Lungs (cont.)

Bronchiectasis	Post-infectious—TB, bacterial or viral pneumonia, recurrent sinus infection Congenital—dyskinetic ciliary syndrome, Kartagener's syndrome, Williams–Campbell syndrome, Mounier–Kuhn syndrome sequestrated lung, cystic fibrosis Obstruction—cancer, TB stenosis, inhaled foreign body Bronchopulmonary aspergillosis Hypogammaglobulin-aemia Chronic aspiration Traction (interstitial fibrosis)
Central bronchiectasis	Allergic bronchopulmonary aspergillosis Cystic fibrosis
Upper lobe fibrosis	TB, histoplasmosis Sarcoid Extrinsic allergic alveolitis (chronic) Radiation Progressive massive fibrosis Ankylosing spondylitis

Lungs (cont.)

CXR air–fluid levels	Lung cavities (see below) Hydropneumothorax Haemopneumo-pericardium Dilated oesophagus Hiatal hernia Chest wall abscess
Diffuse alveolar haemorrhage	Bleeding disorders Any cause of haemoptysis and complicated by aspiration Goodpasture's syndrome SLE Wegener's granulomatosis Systemic vasculitis Drugs Blunt chest trauma Idiopathic pulmonary haemosiderosis
Pulmonary infiltrates with eosinophilia (pulmonary eosinophilia ± blood eosinophilia)	Leoffler's syndrome (simple eosinophilic pneumonia) Chronic eosinophilic pneumonia Acute eosinophilic pneumonia Idiopathic hypereosinophilic syndrome (eosinophilic leukaemia) Churg–Strauss syndrome

Lungs (cont.)

Granulomatous disease	TB, *Mycobacterium avium-intracellulare*
	Sarcoid
	Wegener's granulomatosis
	Lymphomatoid granulomatosis
	Allergic granulomatosis (Churg–Strauss syndrome)
	Bronchocentric granulomatosis
Solitary pulmonary nodule (coin lesion)	Tumours (bronchial cancer, metastasis, adenoma)
	Granuloma, usually tuberculoma
	Hamartoma
	Chest wall lesions— pleural mesothelioma, pleural fibroma, skin tumour, nipple
	Others—rounded pneumonia, rheumatoid nodule, hydatid, haematoma, arteriovenous fistula, paraffinoma, bronchial cyst

Lungs (cont.)

Cavitating lung lesion	Infection—TB, hydatid, pyogenic, fungal
	Tumours—primary or secondary squamous
	Collagen diseases— rheumatoid
	Wegener's disease
	Infarct
	Haematoma
	Progressive massive fibrosis
	Sequestrated segment
	Cystic bronchiectasis
	DD blebs, bullae, pneumatocoele, cystic bronchiectasis
Intracavitary mass	Necrotic carcinoma
	Haematoma
	Fungal ball
	Complicated hydatid cyst
Miliary nodules	Miliary tuberculosis
	Miliary metastases
	Sarcoidosis
	Silicosis
	Fungal diseases— histoplasmosis, coccidiodomycosis

Lungs (cont.)

Small nodular pattern (1–5 mm nodules)	Metastases: • Thyroid, breast, renal Lymphoma Interstitial granulomas: • Sarcoidosis • Chronic hypersensitivity pneumonitis • PLCH • Miliary infections (TB, cryptococcus, coccidioidomycosis and histoplasmosis) • Wegener's granulomatosis • Lymphomatoid granulomatosis Pneumoconiosis: • Silicosis, coal workers' pneumoconiosis, berryllosis and talcosis
Large nodules	Metastases Abscesses Rheumatoid disease Wegener's granulomatosis
Rapidly progressive pulmonary nodules	Fungal pneumonia Septic emboli Tuberculous infection Fulminant metastatic disease Haemorrhagic metastatic disease
Small lungs	Expiration Interstitial fibrosis Bilateral lobar collapse Bilateral elevated diaphragms Obesity Ascites Term pregnancy

Pulmonary oedema

Pulmonary oedema	Heart failure Renal failure Liver failure Aspiration Chest trauma Drug hypersensitivity Drug overdose (heroin) Fluid overload High altitude Inhalation of toxic agents Intracranial disease Near drowning Oxygen toxicity Shock lung Transfusion reaction
Unilateral pulmonary oedema	Prolonged lateral decubitus position Unilateral aspiration Pulmonary contusion Thoracentesis Bronchial obstruction
Hydrostatic pulmonary oedema	Volume overload Renal failure: • Over-hydration Decreased oncotic pressure: • Hypoalbuminaemia Heart disease—'cardiogenic': • Mitral stenosis/regurgitation • Acute myocardial infarction • Acute arrhythmia • Left ventricular aneurysm • Pulmonary veno-occlusive disease

Pulmonary oedema (cont.)

Non-cardiogenic oedema without diffuse alveolar damage	Drug reaction Drug overdose Transfusion reaction Neurogenic: • Head trauma • Seizures • Intracranial haemorrhage • Tumour High altitude Near drowning Aspiration Chest trauma Inhalation of toxic agents Oxygen toxicity
Peribronchial cuffing	Asthma Chronic bronchitis Interstitial pulmonary oedema Viral pneumonia
Kerley B lines	Congestive heart failure Lymphangitic carcinoma *Mycoplasma*, viral and *Pneumocystis carinii* pneumonia Interstitial fibrosis Sarcoid

Pulmonary oedema (cont.)

Diffuse alveolar damage	Idiopathic—acute interstitial pneumonia Risk factors: • Adult respiratory distress syndrome • Sepsis • Shock • Aspiration • Pneumonia • Trauma (direct lung trauma and fat embolism) • Pancreatitis • Radiation • Toxic gas inhalation • Near drowning • Drugs • Transfusional reaction

Bones

Inferior rib notching	Coarctation
	Tetralogy of Fallot (unilateral, usually left side)
	Blalock–Taussig shunt (unilateral right)
	Neurofibromatosis
	Vena caval obstruction
	Pulmonary atresia
Superior rib notching	Quadriplegia
	Poliomyelitis
	Rheumatoid arthritis
	Scleroderma

General

Abnormal air collections	Subcutaneous emphysema
	Pneumothorax
	Pneumomediastinum
	Pulmonary interstitial emphysema
	Lung cavity
	Air embolism

Syndromes relevant to chest radiology

Acute chest syndrome General term used in patients with sickle cell haemoglobinopathy who develop fever and chest symptoms and signs; due to either pneumonia or pulmonary infarction.

Acquired immunodeficiency syndrome (AIDS) Human immuno-deficiency virus (HIV) infection and a CD4$^+$ T lymphocyte count < 200/μL.

Adult respiratory distress syndrome (ARDS) Lung injury characterised by permeability, pulmonary oedema and alveolar damage.

Behçet's disease Chronic relapsing vasculitis secondary to immune complex deposition; also known as Hughes–Stovin syndrome.

Blesovsky syndrome Round atelectasis or folded lung that resembles a mass; can be a consequence of asbestos exposure.

Boerhaave's syndrome Severe vomiting can cause a tear in the oesophageal wall leading to acute mediastinitis.

Caplan's syndrome Pulmonary nodules developing in coal miners with rheumatoid arthritis.

Carney's triad Multiple pulmonary chrondromas, gastric leiomyoblastoma and phaeochromacytoma.

Chung–Strauss syndrome Small vessel vasculitis in patients with asthma and peripheral eosinophilia; also called allergic granulomatosis and angiitis, and allergic granulomatosis.

Ciliary dyskinesia syndrome Impaired mucociliary clearance causes recurrent upper and lower respiratory tract infections. Also known as immobile (immotile) ciliary syndrome.

Congenital pulmonary venolobar syndrome Hypoplastic right lung with a prominent pulmonary vein (scimitar sign) draining into the inferior vena cava. Also known as the hypogenetic lung syndrome and scimitar syndrome.

Dressler's syndrome Fever, pleuritis, pneumonitis and pericarditis occurring a few days or weeks after myocardial infarction. A similar syndrome occurs after cardiac surgery.

Dyskinetic cilia syndrome See Ciliary dyskinesia syndrome.

Ebstein's anomaly Downward displacement of the tricuspid valve into the right ventricle and associated great enlargement of the right atrium.

Ehlos–Danlos syndrome Underlying defect in the elastic tissue; can be complicated by an aortic aneurysm.

Eisenmenger's syndrome Reversal of flow occurring where there is chronic pulmonary hypertension and longstanding left-to-right shunts.

Fallot's tetralogy The primary changes are infundibular stenosis and a high ventricular septal defect. Overriding of the aorta and right ventricular hypertrophy are the secondary structural defects.

Fat embolism syndrome Effects of fat embolism on the lungs and other organs.

Goodpasture's syndrome One of the pulmonary–renal syndromes manifesting as diffuse pulmonary haemorrhage and glomerulo-nephritis.

Hamman–Rich syndrome Acute interstitial pneumonia.

Hantavirus pulmonary syndrome Infection with the hantavirus causes severe damage to pulmonary capillary endothelium with consequential pulmonary oedema of the increased permeability type.

Horner's syndrome Eye signs. Local ipsilateral destruction of the sympathetic chain by a Pancoast tumour.

Hughes–Stovin syndrome See Behçet's disease.

Hypogenetic lung syndrome Hypoplastic right lung with anomalous pulmonary vein draining into the inferior vena cava. Also known as congenital pulmonary venolobar syndrome and scimitar syndrome.

Kartagener's syndrome Situs inversus (dextrocardia), bronchiectasis and sinusitis.

Klippel–Trenauney–Weber syndrome Numerous arteriovenous malformations which can involve the chest wall.

Lady Windermere syndrome Non-tuberculous mycobacterial infection occurring in patients without underlying lung disease. These patients are usually elderly females who have an irritating chronic cough. A 'tree-in-bud' appearance is seen on HRCT, mainly occurring in the right middle lobe and lingular segment.

Loeffler's syndrome Patchy migratory infiltrates on CXR due to an allergic reaction to parasitic infiltration of lungs.

MacLeod's syndrome Acquired hypoplasia of one lung secondary to infantile obliterative bronchiolitis; consequential small pulmonary artery and bronchiectasis. Also known as Swyer–James syndrome.

Marfan's syndrome Connective disease disorder; predisposed to aortic aneurysms and dissections.

Meig's syndrome Non-neoplastic pleural effusion and ascites associated with a benign ovarian tumour (a malignant ovarian tumour needs to be excluded). Also known as Meig–Salmon syndrome.

Mendelson's syndrome Aspiration of gastric contents.

Middle lobe syndrome Chronic and recurrent collapse of the right middle lobe.

Mounier–Kuhn syndrome Tracheobronchomegaly.

Organic dust toxic syndrome Exposure to organic dusts can cause an influenza-like symptom complex.

Pancoast syndrome Symptom complex of pain in the shoulder or arm from an apical tumour invading the brachial plexus and sympathetic chain.

Pickwickian syndrome Morbidly obese with alveolar hypo-ventilation and pulmonary hypertension.

Poland syndrome Congenital defect of the pectoral muscle.

Rendu–Osler–Weber syndrome Hereditary haemorrhagic telangiectasia with multiple arteriovenous malformations.

Riley–Day syndrome Hereditary neurological disease with dysplasia and recurrent episodes of aspiration bronchopneumonia; consequential bronchiectasis.

Severe acute respiratory syndrome (SARS) Influenza-like infection caused by a coronavirus.

Scimitar syndrome Also known as congenital pulmonary venolobar syndrome and hypogenetic lung syndrome.

Sjögren's syndrome Polyarthritis with dry mucous membranes; also known as sicca syndrome.

Tropical eosinophilia Episodic cough and wheezing, high blood eosinophilia and diffuse reticulonodular infiltrates on the chest radiograph.

Vanishing lung syndrome Markedly progressive emphysema with giant bullae.

Williams–Campbell syndrome Tracheobronchomalacia.

Wilson–Mikity syndrome A form of pulmonary dysmaturity in premature neonates which differs from bronchopulmonary dysplasia in that there is no history of hyaline membrane disease, prolonged oxygen therapy or mechanical ventilation.

Yellow nail syndrome A triad of yellow nails, pleural effusion and primary lymphoedema. Other respiratory manifestations include recurrent bronchitis, pneumonia, pleurisy, bronchiectasis and sinusitis.

Index

References to figures and tables are in *italics*.